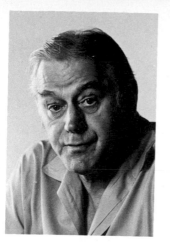

About the author:

PAUL ENGLE is known to many for a variety
of reasons. The director of the University
of Iowa Writers' Workshop for twenty-five
years, he and his wife, Hualing Nieh,
founded the UI International Writing Pro-
gram in 1966. He has authored twelve volumes of poetry, one of which was awarded
the Yale Series of Younger Poets prize. He
has a published novel and two nonfiction
books to his credit, as well as articles in
many periodicals, among them *Ladies'
Home Journal, The New Yorker, Saturday
Evening Post,* and *Harper's.* Mr. Engle has
traveled extensively throughout the world
and has lectured at numerous universities
and clubs. A Rhodes scholar, he has also
been awarded grants from the Ford, Rocke-
feller, and Guggenheim foundations and is
at this time a candidate with his wife for
the 1976 Nobel Prize for Peace. He has done
research on women in American history,
from the beginning of the 17th century to
1890, and will publish further books in the
field. Paul Engle presently resides in Iowa
City with his wife, a writer and scholar born
in mainland China, and her two children.

Women in the
American Revolution

Women in the American Revolution

By PAUL ENGLE

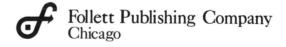

Follett Publishing Company
Chicago

Contents

List of Illustrations

Acknowledgments

Many librarians (they must be the most unrewarded people on earth) generously helped with this book. Jean Wylder began it all some years ago with diligent and insightful research. John Abel worked strenuously on many of the chapters and provided a central point of view. Wayne Prophet, Tom Zynda, Michael Veitch, Diane Powell, and Kathleen Welch all contributed. The Graduate College of the University of Iowa supported some of the research. The dean of the college, Duane Spriestersbach, has been most sympathetic. Merilyn Munneke provided invaluable assistance.

The historical societies of all the states represented in this book answered queries and provided bibliographical data.

Ada Stoflet, Reference Department, University of Iowa Library, was not only able but indispensable, as always.

Mary Burge of Cambridge, Massachusetts, supplied additional information, advice, and her knowledge of American literature and history.

A remarkable Chinese lady, Hualing Nieh Engle, made me aware of what it is to be a woman and an American.

Introduction

THE FIRST 150 years of colonial life in America, beginning with the clearing of trees along the desolate shores of the Atlantic, required such enormous endurance, resolution, and fortitude, that they left an indelible stamp on a people that marked them American, not English, and made the Revolutionary War inevitable.

They had survived the test of time and climate and great hardship, had built a country by hand, and so had come to an age of wisdom and independence. The rigors of colonial life created a rich testing ground particularly for the women. Unlike their European counterparts who moved within a fixed, stable society, American women had to share the total new experience. If they lived in deep forests, they knew how to handle an axe; if they lived on the banks of rivers, they knew how to handle boats. They defended their homes and children from Indian attacks and the harshness of winter. When the Revolution came, they were able to ride horses many miles and handle guns. They recognized death's face staring through the windows and its footsteps shuffling down the trails behind them. Disaster had walked hand in hand with them, for many died early from overwork and too frequent childbearing. However, they all contributed overwhelmingly to the taming of a wild country.

Almost from the start women had a stake in the land: they sometimes owned it in all of the colonies; they worked it and were responsible for its management. Eliza Lucas, still in her teens, managed three plantations during her father's absence, besides devoting herself to music and gardening. To her, South Carolina owed the introduction of the important crop of indigo, which she cultivated from seed, experimenting and refining the process until by 1746 it had become the most valuable Carolina export. In letters written to her father in 1742, we find that she was creating ". . .a large plantation of oaks which I look upon as my own property . . . and therefore I design many years hence when oaks are more valuable than they are now, which you know they will be when we come to build fleets. . . ." In that same year she had planted a large fig orchard with the idea of exporting the dried fruit. "I love the vegitable world extreamly," she added, but assured her father that she still had time for beaux and the pleasures offered by the town.

Before the Revolution women owned and managed profitable businesses. Flora Dorsey kept the Lover Ferry on the Ptapsco River in Maryland for twenty-five years. In 1753 Hannah Dubre announced in the Philadelphia press that she sold all sorts of seeds and did so for the next fifteen years. Women advertised their products in the colonial newspapers regularly: Hannah Moses sold trinkets in Philadelphia; Mary Salmon of Boston and Mrs. Proctor of Salem shoed horses. On March 28, 1748 Hannah Chapman advertised in the *Boston Evening Post* that she "makes and sells a Smell in Mixture, that will cure the Itch or any other breaking out, by the Smell of it."

Women not only advertised their wares and businesses in the newspapers, they also ran newspapers and printing businesses, taking over at their husbands' deaths. Anything men could do as newspaper publishers, women could do also, and as well, and sometimes better. There were a few newspapers that espoused the early cause of free speech and liberty, among them the *Maryland Gazette* which was suspended on account of the Stamp Act in 1765. The publisher's widow, Anne Katherine Green, started the paper up again in 1767, putting out the first copies as *The Apparition of the Maryland Gazette Which Is not Dead But Sleepth.* Instead of a stamp, it bore a death's head with the motto, "The times are Dismal, Doleful, Dolorous, Dollarless." Anne Katherine carried on the paper until 1775, with occasional assistance from her son. Likewise, Anna Zenger had a hand in her husband's *New York Weekly Journal* which openly criticized King George and the Loyalist contingent that governed the colonies. Kent Cooper* maintains that it was Anna who wrote the anonymous satirical articles on the English

Anna Zenger, The Mother of Freedom (New York: Farrar, Straus & Giroux, Inc., 1946).

government and not her husband John Peter Zenger, who may have been barely literate. Anna ran an ad in the *Journal* after his death in 1747 " . . . to acquaint the Public that some Evil minded Persons have been pleased to spread a Report abroad that the Widow Zenger, Publisher of this Paper, had entirely dropped the Printing Business, etc. This is therefore to give notice, that the said Report is Notoriously False, and that the said Widow still continues the Printing Business, where any Person may have their work done reasonable, in a good Manner, and with Expedition."

Mary Beard points out that in all great upheavals in history women have responded as activists and thinkers. American colonial women during the Revolution were no exception—they were ready in body and spirit for the independence of the colonies. There were no schools for girls until after the Revolution, but most women had learned to read and write from tutors or their fathers or husbands. Now they were to write letters to arouse anyone they suspected of lagging and to communicate information.

The first news of the Boston Tea Party was probably Abigail Adams's comment in her letter to Mercy Warren: "You, madam, are so sincere a lover of your country, and so hearty a mourner in all her misfortunes, that it will greatly aggravate your anxiety to hear how much she is now oppressed and insulted. . . . The tea, that baneful weed, is arrived: great, and I hope effectual opposition has been made to the landing."

The war took place in backyards, in gardens, down the street, in the cow pasture, behind barns, around rural taverns (with a shattering loss of bottles), in tobacco fields, over stands of wheat. In short, in every place where women lived and worked. Thus, women were given their first opportunity to unite their efforts for a great common cause beyond the scope of their town or farm. In the early stages they were quick to organize themselves into the Daughters of Liberty: they set up day-long sewing meetings in order to supply the markets with goods that had been closed off to importation; they boycotted anything British with unrelenting vigor; and they cheered on the crowds that tore down royal insignia. In North Carolina the young women vowed not to "date" any man who had not been in service.

Wherever women lived, they contributed to the war effort. When word reached Connecticut that fighting had begun, Ruth Draper baked brown bread for two days and a night, getting some of her neighbors to do the same. By the time hundreds of troops began to pass by her farm, she had enough bread and cheese and cider ready on long roadside tables to feed them. After Bunker Hill had depleted ammunition supplies, Washington issued a call for every ounce of lead or pewter available. The same Mrs. Draper turned in all her pewter plates, pans, and dishes—heirlooms brought to America by her English ancestors were now used to make bullets to fire at the British.

In Charleston, South Carolina, Mrs. Sabina Elliott knitted socks for the Americans—some of them with the date 1776 knit in the threads still exist. During the occupation of Charleston by the British, her daughter Ann wore a bonnet decorated with thirteen small plumes to indicate she was a Patriot. She was so beautiful that an English officer offered to defect to the American side if she would have him. She would not, she said, and only scorned a man capable of betraying his sovereign for selfish interest.

In Rhode Island General Greene's wife, Catherine, gave up her house so that it might be used as a hospital for inoculations against smallpox for hundreds of troops and went to share the privations of the long winter at Valley Forge.

In North Carolina Sarah Dickinson, the mother of nine children, saw her plantation laid waste in revenge for her capture of five Loyalists, as was the plantation of Flora M'Donald who had encouraged the Loyalists by marching along with them. Catherine Schuyler is perhaps the best-known of the women who sacrificed their homes for the Patriot cause. The brave wife of Major General Philip Schuyler burned the wide wheat fields of her own estate near Saratoga so that the approaching British—who were running low on food—could not use the grain. When the British General Burgoyne arrived at the abandoned estate, he burned the manor house and other buildings. The senselessness of this act should have infuriated Catherine Schuyler. Yet upon Burgoyne's surrender to the Patriots, the humane Catherine and her husband invited the defeated general to be a guest in their other home near Albany. Was it the unique American experience that gave persons such as Catherine Schuyler the courage to defy all fear, and the generosity to forgive all rudeness?

When Washington lost New York, Abigail Adams wrote John: "We are in no wise dispirited here. We possess a spirit that will not be conquered. If our men are all drawn off and we should be attacked, you would find a race of Amazons in America." She concluded that if the American men surrendered to Howe, "an army of women would oppose him [John]," reminding him that the Saracens were killed by their women when the men turned tail and ran from the foe.

Throughout the war, women collected money for soldiers' equipment or relief. One such association was headed by Esther Reed in Philadelphia in 1780. Hundreds of women from all ranks of society—from Phillis, an old colored woman who gave seven shillings and sixpence to the Countess de Luzerne, who gave $6,000 in continental paper—joined in the common effort until the desired sum had been raised. If they had no money, they made soldiers' shirts; if they gave money, they also gave time to sewing. George Washington, with whom Mrs. Reed corresponded on the best way to distribute the clothing, said she "writes as judiciously on the humble topic of soldiers' shirts, as on the plan of a campaign or the subsistence of an Army."

Every day women went to the hospitals to care for the sick and wounded; they went to the battlefields to look for the wounded and dead; they buried friends and even enemies. American prisoners waited for the women to bring them food. Women kept the farms going while the plowmen were on the battlefront—they raised grain, harvested it, and made bread to carry to their relatives in the army or the prisons. Their spinning wheels and looms went night and day.

Other women are known to have taken up arms on the battlefield. There was Rebecca Motte of South Carolina who, after her plantation house was occupied by the British, helped the Patriots shoot flaming arrows on the roof to burn it down and force a British surrender. At Fort Henry, Virginia, on September 11, 1782, Elizabeth Zane saved the fort and the day by dashing sixty yards to a nearby house for more gunpowder and returning safely in a hail of bullets. Nancy Hart in Georgia, called "War Woman" respectfully by the Indians, killed six Loyalists when they forced their way into her home. Less than a hundred years later during the Civil War, women of Georgia united their forces as the "Nancy Harts" in remembrance of her bravery.

Deborah Sampson Gannett masqueraded as a man long enough to serve in a Massachusetts regiment of the Continental army. She was wounded twice, yet not detected. An illness ended her disguise, but George Washington gave her an honorable discharge, and she became the first woman granted a pension (eight dollars a month) by the U.S. Government.

Molly Pitcher is a legendary figure. There is no clear evidence to prove that Molly was one real person; many feel that she is the embodiment of several individuals who performed heroic actions on the battlefield. We believe that she probably did exist. She is said to have been accompanying her husband's regiment when it faced Clinton at the battle of Monmouth in 1778. The day was a scorching one, and many soldiers collapsed from the heat. The valiant Molly brought water to the men throughout the battle, all the while exposing herself to British fire. For this deed she was dubbed Molly "Pitcher" by the grateful soldiers. She also rescued and nursed wounded men. Finally, when her own husband was felled by the enemy, she took charge of firing his cannon and carried on until the end of the battle. Though she spent the next seven years in the army and performed heroic deeds, Molly was never given a special pension.

Paul Revere's horse is more widely pictured in American history than many real women who also rode in the Patriot cause. Some of them rode farther than he did, in nights as dark and in equal danger. Yet there is little graphic evidence of the young girls and wives who went off on their own—in their long dresses, on back roads, and through wildernesses—to warn Continental soldiers of the British; sometimes their own husbands were in those troops.

On April 26, 1777, sixteen-year-old Sybil Ludington rode forty miles to warn militiamen that the British were marching to burn the Patriot base at Danbury, Connecticut. She rode from the present Ludingtonville, New York, east to Danbury. The militiamen rallied and intercepted the British troops at Ridgefield, but were unable to keep them from breaking through to the south and the Royal Navy ships waiting in Long Island Sound.

There were other women in every one of the colonies who took their lives in their hands, put their lives in the saddle, and trusted their lives to their feet—some of them, over and over again. Kate Moore Barry in South Carolina often acted as a messenger and helped alert the militia for the crucial battle of Cowpens. Grace and Rachel Martin, also of South Carolina, once dressed themselves in men's clothes to waylay a courier accompanied by two British officers. They took the men by surprise at night along a lonely road, obtained important papers, and hurried them to General Greene's camp. In the same colony, Jane Thomas galloped sixty miles to warn a group of Patriots, one of whom was her own son, that a gang of Loyalists was moving to attack them. The ride, much longer than

Paul Revere's, enabled the local boys to organize a defense and defeat the British when they came. It took a tough woman to endure the jolts and friction of sixty miles in a saddle; every inch of that distance might have brought the enemy and capture, if not death. It took not only a firm hand on the reins and a strong foot in the stirrup, but a deep conviction in the mind to perform such triumphs. Throughout the years of the Revolution women rode, walked, and took boats to alert their side to danger from the other.

After the war, the women took a strong part in helping to bring the country back together again, realizing that an end to Loyalist and Patriot bitterness was essential to the continuation of independence. The best example of this role comes from the letter of a woman who had been on the side of the Loyalists. She is the aforementioned Eliza Lucas Pinckney who had, as a teenager, managed her father's estates.

> . . . Both my Sons, their wives and Infants were exiled. . . . Their estates had been long before sequestered and mine was shattered and ruined, which left me little power to assist them; nor had I in Country or Town a place to lay my head, all was taken out of my possession; my house I live in, that in Colleton Square, and at Belmont, all was taken from me, nor was I able to hire a lodging. But let me forget as soon as I can their cruelties, I wish to forgive and will say no more on this subject, and hope our joy and gratitude for our great deliverance may equal our former anguish, and our contentment in mediocrity, and moderation in prosperity, equal the fortitude with which the greatest number even of our sex sustained the great reverse of fortune they experienced. . . .

The war had been everywhere, as had been women of every temperament, appearance, degree of intelligence and education. There was not one of the colonies in which women had not taken an active part, even if it were only in the sewing of many hundreds of shirts for the soldiers. For it had been their war, too, not merely their men's.

PART I

Battlefield Heroines

1

Dicey Langston

DICEY LANGSTON was born Laodicea in 1760 on her father's plantation in South Carolina. Their home was in the Laurens District on the Enoree River. Dicey's mother died when she was still a little girl, and under the tutelage of her two brothers, she grew up a tomboy—sharing their life and learning their games and skills.

When the Revolution broke out, she was only sixteen, but like her brothers she was a Patriot and she made this clear to everyone. She could ride a horse and handle a rifle as expertly as they could. Her father Solomon shared his children's zeal for independence, but he was an old man now. He could not take the part of a fighter in the field, but he could and did help the Patriots whenever he could with money and influence. He was a planter, and he had not only his family's safety to worry about, but he also had to guard his property against the predations of the Loyalists, who far outnumbered the Patriots in the Laurens District.

The other people in the area knew about Solomon Langston's sons who had taken up their rifles and gone into the field as soldiers as soon as the war broke out. Staying away from the family plantation to protect it against Loyalist reprisals, they camped out along the Enoree several miles from home. What people did not know for a while was that Dicey kept in constant touch with her brothers. She was their link of communication with the plantation and also, as the Loyalists eventually discovered, with themselves. At first, however, she appeared to them only as the lovely and sweet young daughter of an old planter.

The war in the South had an important difference from the war in the North. This difference made life much harder for Southern Patriots and Loyalists alike, and especially for the women of the families.

The North was a country of towns. The produce of its farms went to feed the towns and the cities which were centers of the import-export trade. The Stamp Act, the Navigation Acts, and the Townshend Acts were, therefore, resented as intolerable oppressions. The towns were generally pro-independence, so that the Loyalists, who were often outnumbered, were hounded and harassed. In some towns Loyalists were hanged, or beaten, or tarred and feathered—this was a severe punishment, for they had no way to get the tar off—or run out of town without a means of survival. Those who refused to take up arms, whether for reasons of politics or conscience, were maltreated and abused and sometimes simply taken to the town square and shot. Yet, at least the towns served as centers of opinion; each had a certain political orientation that was enforced by social, political, and economic pressure.

The sympathies of the town were not always ironclad, however. When the British occupied Philadelphia, there were many inhabitants who refused to fraternize with the troops, but the colonists did not try to kill other townspeople who did. Many Philadelphians enjoyed a glittering social life with the British officers and did a lucrative business with the British army. In the meantime, thirty miles away at Valley Forge, Washington's men were starving and shivering because they couldn't match the British ability to pay high prices for food and cloth.

The South was totally different. In this expansive land, life was organized around the plantations rather than around the towns. The plantations were large and the families, therefore, were widely separated; political opinion could vary like night and day from one plantation to the next, even in the same area.

Overall, the South was more Loyalist in sentiment than the North. The planters depended on Britain not only as a market for their tobacco, but also for the ships to get it to market and the naval power to protect the ships' cargoes. The British laws, so oppressive to the commercial North, did not bother the planters. They had a vested interest in the stability of British rule and a great deal to lose if the Revolution succeeded.

In the South differences of opinion caused great bitterness. This region became involved not only in the Revolution against Britain, but also in a simultaneous civil war among its own people. Both sides formed guerrilla bands that fought without the rules that governed and tempered the violence of the legitimate armies. These small bands attacked each other, raided plantations and settlements, and destroyed property and crops. Often the Loyalist bands included men who had been malcontents or plain outlaws before the war and who now found some status and power in fighting for the British. They could also settle their personal grudges under the guise of fighting as soldiers. Victory was achieved not by taking and holding a town, but by destroying or taking over a plantation and killing its owner and his family.

The plantations were more vulnerable to attack than the towns of the North. A town could return considerable fire to anyone attacking it; while a plantation house could be surprised at night by a small band, its few defenders shot (even if they were awake), and the house looted. Defense against the guerrillas was difficult, for there was no way to get help from sympathetic neighbors. The first news one would have of an attack on a neighbor was likely to be the plume of smoke from a burning house, or the arrival of survivors in need of aid. Then the revenge of one's own side would be plotted.

The Laurens District was notoriously dangerous for Patriots. Some of Dicey's own relatives were Loyalists, and she and her father and brothers were the political enemies of the relatives with whom they had Sunday dinner. However, this was a means by which Dicey gained information regarding Loyalist activities and plans. During visits she simply listened to the conversations for any news of enemy moves, and since the war was the biggest topic of conversation, she heard a great deal. Later she would go off to find her brothers' camp and report the information to them.

Dicey's relatives considered her only a child, and they made no attempt to hide their conversations from her. After a while, though, when they wondered how news of their plans seemed to constantly make its way to the Patriot bands, they became suspicious of her. Other Loyalists in the area who hated the Langstons for their political sympathies knew of Dicey's contact with her Loyalist relatives and decided to take action.

At first they only threatened. They warned Solomon to put a stop to Dicey's spying or else suffer the consequences himself. Solomon had to depend on the restraint of his Loyalist neighbors for the safety of Dicey's life, his own life, and his property; therefore, he agreed to their ultimatum. He forbade Dicey to pass any more information to her brothers, and she—as an obedient daughter who did not want to give her old father worry, much less place him in danger—agreed to his order.

However, her retirement from active duty lasted only a few

weeks. One of the Loyalist bands operating in the Laurens District was called the Bloody Scouts; their name describes the ruthless cruelty that marked their raids on defenseless families living on isolated plantations and settlements. Dicey learned that the Bloody Scouts were going to attack a small Patriot settlement called Little Eden, located near her brothers' camp.

Dicey knew that the settlement would be taken by surprise; the people would not have time to get together a defense; and at least some of them would be murdered. Moreover, in the attack on Little Eden, the Bloody Scouts would certainly find her brothers' camp and kill them.

Dicey had to get word to them of the Bloody Scouts' plans, but she could not let her father find out because of the promise she had made to him. She knew, too, that if her father knew, he might be forced to admit it to Loyalists who questioned him, and above all she had to keep the Loyalists from finding out. The slightest suspicion would bring them down on her father; they hated him and were anxious for an excuse to kill him and take his property. She had no one whom she could trust to send to give warning. If her brothers and Little Eden were to be saved, she must go herself. She must go at night, and she must go on foot, since taking a horse would not only rouse the household but also make her a target for Loyalist gangs on the road.

When everyone in the house was asleep that night, she set off alone and on foot. She stayed away from the roads because they were haunted by Loyalist gangs. Dicey went through woods and fields, even where there were no paths to follow, with only her sense of direction to lead her. She made steady progress until she came to a swollen and rushing creek; there was no bridge or even a log to take her across. She did not know how deep the water was, but to deliver her warning she had to get to the other bank; she decided to take her chances and ford the creek. The swift current made her lose her footing on the mud bottom, and the water picked her up and spun her around as it carried her downstream. When she finally regained her footing against the current, she could not tell which bank she had stepped from and which she had to get to. Trusting her instinct, she climbed the bank and set off in the direction she thought led to her brothers' camp.

Her instinct had been right! After hours of hiking she came to the camp. The men had just returned from a mission, and they were tired, wet, and hungry. She gave them the news of the Bloody

Scouts' plans, but they were all too exhausted to set off to warn the settlers. She saw that nothing could be done until they had food.

She had them build a fire. Although she, too, was exhausted and wet, she made a hoecake from the flour and cornmeal they had on hand. She spread the dough on a board and laid it in the embers of the fire to bake. In a short time the hoecake was ready and the men made plans. They each took some of the bread in their ammunition pouches to eat on the way and set off to warn the settlers.

The Bloody Scouts rode down on Little Eden at the first light of morning and found it completely empty.

While the gang boiled with rage over the frustration of their plan, Dicey was back at the plantation, freshly dressed and having breakfast with her family. She had made a twenty-mile trip through the night, and she was so tired she could hardly converse. Her father wondered if she was ill, but he did not suspect her nighttime adventures.

The frustration of the Bloody Scouts in missing so easy a target as Little Eden added fuel to their hatred of the few Patriots in the Laurens District. They began again to focus their suspicions and dislike on Langston and his daughter. When Dicey's brothers joined with some other Patriots in an attack on local Loyalists, the Bloody Scouts decided to make Langston their next target.

They came ready to kill him. The household was defenseless, and considering Solomon's infirm condition, he and Dicey could not even escape.

The Loyalist leader demanded to know from Langston what part he had had in raids on members of their group. When he denied having any active part, the leader accused him of lying. The Loyalist leader pointed his pistol at Solomon's heart and cocked it; Dicey jumped between her father and the pistol and began harshly denouncing the gunman, who became so angry that he nearly shot her instead. One of the guerrillas got his leader under control. He had been fully ready to see Solomon shot, but he felt that killing Dicey was going too far. The Loyalists got into an argument among themselves, and their enthusiasm for finishing off Solomon was lost in the quarreling. They left as angry as when they had forced their way inside but with their nerve broken by Dicey's defiance.

The raid on the house did not mark the end of the gang's harassment of the Langstons. Not long afterward Dicey ran into the gang as she was heading homeward from the Spartansburg District.

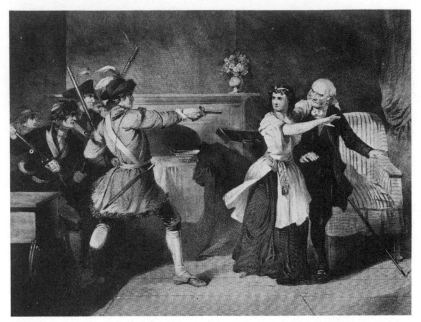

*Dicey Langston shielding her father. (Engraving by Alfred Jones)
Courtesy, Historical Pictures Service, Chicago*

They saw her coming and blocked the road; though she was a skillful rider, she had no choice but to halt and face them. The leader demanded to know what news she had of the Patriots. She explained that she had seen none on her visit, and so she had no news to give him even if she were willing to. He held his pistol to her chest and gave her one last chance to tell him what she knew. To this, Dicey pulled open the front of her riding habit and dared him to fire! The enraged Loyalist was about to pull the trigger when one of his own men reached out and knocked the leader's arm upward, and the bullet sailed off into the sky instead of into Dicey. His attempted murder sabotaged by his own follower, his pistol empty and his nerve rattled, the leader forgot about Dicey and attacked the man who had saved her. The other guerrillas joined in the fight and forgot about Dicey. She gave her horse a lash and took off down the road at a full gallop toward her home.

Just as the Loyalists had finally learned to treat Dicey with the respect due an equal opponent, the Patriots had also gained some sharp awakenings as to the pugnacity of the deceptively ingenuous young girl. One Patriot leader learned the hard way—by getting the treatment she usually reserved for Loyalists—not to take Dicey for granted.

This Patriot leader had come to the Langston plantation to pick up a rifle which one of Dicey's brothers had left with her. The latter had told her that she would recognize the man by a countersign he would give her. The Patriot and his band explained to Dicey that they were friends of her brother and had been instructed to get the rifle from her. Dicey retrieved the rifle from its hiding place, but as she was about to turn it over, she hesitated. The band was suspicious looking. She thought they might well be Loyalists since she had never seen any of them before. To make sure, she asked the leader for the countersign. The leader laughed and told her that it was too late for that sort of thing since he now had both the rifle and herself in his possession. His teasing was cut short in a moment; Dicey cocked the rifle and pointed it at him, inviting him to try and take what he thought he had. In a chilling instant he realized she meant it; he gave her the countersign and later bore the laughter of his men for being tripped up by the girl. He and Dicey must have been impressed with each other though—after the war she married him.

Dicey was not so fanatical a Patriot that she only judged persons by their politics; she was more concerned with the human qualities of the people she knew. One of her neighbors was another planter whom Dicey liked, though he was a Loyalist. He was a good man and a friend of the Langstons, and his Loyalist sympathies did not lead him to violence. Dicey was serving food to a group of her brothers' friends who had stopped at the house when she heard that they were on their way to steal this neighbor's horses. He would be an easy target, and the Patriots could certainly use the horses. But Dicey did not want to see her neighbor injured—he'd done nothing to deserve it, and it would cause bitterness between him and the Langstons.

While the Patriots talked over their plans, Dicey excused herself and ran to the neighbor's house to warn him that his horses were in danger. As she was leaving, she overheard someone say that word of the Patriot band had been sent to a Loyalist gang in the area. She ran back to her house where, fortunately, the Patriots were still eating and talking, and warned them of the danger. She had saved the neighbor's horses, but she also saved the lives of her friends.

Harassment by the Loyalists continued throughout the war, and with her brothers in the field, Dicey was all that stood between the household and the Loyalist gangs. Sometimes she was able to get rid of the armed gangs through sheer nerve: she would refuse to open the door, shout and threaten, and they would eventually leave. Sometimes she was not so successful, and the gang would break in and steal what they wanted. Usually, she won out.

After the war Thomas Springfield, the Patriot leader whom she had taught not to tease her, came back to the plantation to court her. She married him and went to Greenville where she lived to a very advanced age. She was particularly proud of the large number of sons and grandsons she had, for they could all vote as free men.

2

Lydia Darragh

DURING THE REVOLUTION the British often took over private homes for the use of their army in areas they occupied. This was not a matter of malice or a special technique of oppression, but simply standard practice for armies in the eighteenth century. The homes were used for housing officers, as meeting places, and as mess halls.

Fairly early in the war, Philadelphia, the city where the First and Second Continental Congresses had met and where the Constitution was drawn up, was taken and occupied by the British in September 1777.

Lydia Darragh's home in Philadelphia was on Second Street near Spruce, just a block from the wharves and across the street from the Golden Fleece Tavern—and it was also across the street from General Howe's headquarters. Howe requisitioned one of the rooms in her house for the use of his officers on the advice of Lydia's own cousin, a lieutenant in the British army. This was Howe's undoing, for the use of Lydia's house led to his defeat in what otherwise would have been a victory over Washington's forces.

Lydia was not a native Philadelphian. She was born Lydia Barrington in 1729 in Dublin. The Barringtons kept a clergyman's son, one William Darragh, as a tutor for the children. During this student-tutor relationship, William and Lydia fell in love, and late in 1753 William married his twenty-four-year-old sweetheart. They were Quakers, and very soon after their marriage the couple emigrated to Philadelphia. Though she was a small woman and her friends thought her "very delicate in appearance," she took up the backbreaking occupation of nurse and midwife, and in 1766 she even established a mortuary.

Lydia's work provided the main support for her family. Her husband did not earn much as a teacher, and they had nine children to raise. Her reputation for tenderness and ability in nursing made her a good provider for the family, and she was able to rent a large house.

When the Revolution came, Lydia was already outspokenly and actively pro-American, even to the point of violating the pacifism she was committed to as a Quaker. She became a "Fighting Quaker"—one of a group of persons who retained their faith while taking part in the war. Although Lydia herself did not fire a cannon, her son Charles became an officer in the Continental army and, as we shall see, she did everything she could to help Washington's forces.

On December 2, 1777—two months after Philadelphia had been taken—Howe's adjutant came to her house and told her that the officers would be using a room for a meeting at seven o'clock that evening. He also told her that he wanted the family to be asleep early for the privacy of the officers.

Lydia felt that the adjutant was being unusually careful; obviously this was not a routine conference. She sent her family to bed early, let the officers into the house, and went to her room—but she did not go to sleep. She got up, crept to the door of the conference room, put her ear to the keyhole, and listened.

She heard an officer reading an order for all British troops to march out of the city on the night of the fourth to attack Washington's forces at Whitemarsh, a town north of Philadelphia.

While they were getting ready to leave, she hurried back to her room and climbed into bed. Soon the officers came to wake her to let them out of the house; she let them knock three times before she opened the door, causing them to think she must have been in deep sleep.

Lydia could not sleep that night. She knew that if she could somehow get her information to Washington in time, she would save a large number of American lives. She also knew that the British would hang her if they found out.

The next day, without telling even her husband of what she knew or of her true errand, she announced that she had to go to Frankford—outside the city—for flour. She went across the street to General Howe and asked for a pass through the British lines to get to the flour mill. Suspecting nothing, Howe complied immediately.

With a flour sack over her shoulder, Lydia set out to ruin Howe's plans.

She actually did go to the flour mill at Frankford, but there she left her bag of flour and set off to find the American lines.

Whitemarsh was only thirteen miles from Philadelphia. Washington had a large force of his own troops there, along with about 2,200 more from Rhode Island, Maryland, and Pennsylvania as reinforcements. At this point he was hoping for a battle with Howe, but he did not want to engage him until he was sure he was in a position to win a decisive victory. With this in mind he did not group his troops for an attempt to retake Philadelphia, but instead he used them to harass the British general. By a resolution of the Continental Congress, any person found within a thirty-mile radius of a place held by the British, in the act of carrying supplies to them, was to be arrested and held under martial law. Washington had his troops out in small squads patroling the roads around the city, checking on the movement of people and supplies, and looking for such collaborators. This gave him two advantages, for he not only caused Howe a great deal of trouble by denying him supplies by land, but he also increased his own provisions by confiscating any he found bound for the British.

As Lydia walked along the road toward Washington's lines, she ran into one of his patrols. By luck the officer in charge was a man she knew, a friend of her brother. She talked with him for a while, receiving news of her brother. Since she could not reveal herself to the whole squad as a spy, she asked the officer to leave his horse and walk with her so that they could speak privately. She made him first promise not to identify her as the source of his information, for she had herself and her family to protect; then she told him of the British plans. The officer took her to a house nearby, asked the woman there to feed Lydia, and then galloped to General Washington with her news.

Lydia ate and rested awhile, returned to the mill to pick up her flour, and walked back through the British lines to her home. The next days were anxious ones for her, since she had to conceal her act not only from the British, but from everyone else as well. Still thinking that they had the supreme advantage of surprise, the British marched out on the night of December 4 as planned, and Lydia alone knew that what awaited them was what they least expected. Her anxiety involved more than just keeping this secret. If

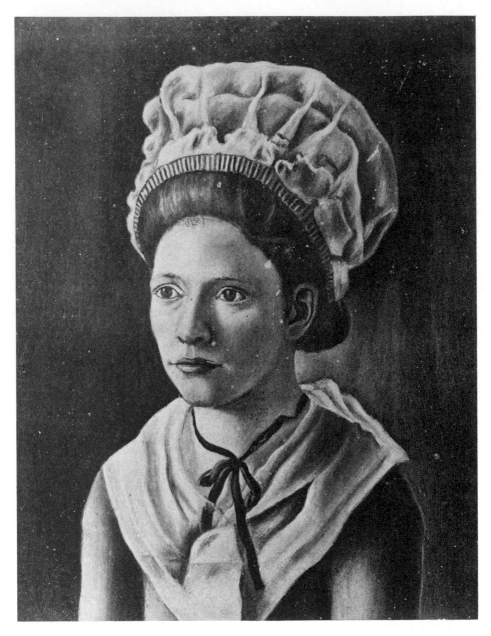

Lydia Darragh (presumed portrait)
Courtesy, Frick Art Reference Library

Washington had not used her information to prepare for the attack, the British would kill many Americans. On the other hand, if he were ready for them, the British would suspect her and she might be killed.

On the eighth the British returned dejected. They had accomplished nothing, much less a victory over the Continentals. Washington had been ready for them.

For the troops on both sides, the ordeal was over; they had won or lost, been wounded, killed, or spared—but it was over. For Lydia, the most trying experience was yet to come, for now the British would suspect her as the cause of their defeat.

The evening after the troops returned, Howe's adjutant came again, only this time he took the terrified Lydia into a room and locked the door. He questioned her about the family—had anyone not been in bed? Could anyone have listened at the door? He could think of no other explanation for the fiasco that had befallen his troops. Despite his pressure, Lydia remained perfectly calm. She explained that everyone had been in bed and asleep by eight o'clock, and she was sure no one had gotten up to eavesdrop. The adjutant accepted her explanation, which indeed was true as far as it went. There was only Lydia left for him to consider, but he saved her the trouble of having to lie convincingly, for he told her that he knew she had been asleep since it had taken him so long to wake her when the meeting ended. The adjutant had to leave without finding a culprit to hang, and the British did not bother her about the matter after this. Lydia's plot had succeeded, and she had escaped without being discovered.

This was not the last of Lydia's efforts to help the Continentals, although it was the most dangerous—she could easily have lost her life. Nothing suggests that her cousin, Lieutenant Barrington, would have or could have done anything to save her had Howe discovered her exploit. Lydia continued aiding the cause of independence, going out from Philadelphia to nurse the refugees from the city who lived in the surrounding area.

Lydia's hard and competent work as a nurse and midwife had given her a fine reputation. In addition, she kept a small store in her home, and despite the demands of her large family she was prosperous. Her husband left her a substantial estate when he died in 1783, and a few years later she was able to purchase the house on Second Street where her daring exploit had begun.

At about the same time, however, she was troubled in other

aspects of her life. In 1783 the monthly meeting of Friends suspended her for neglecting to attend its meetings and for "ignoring the admonitions of her fellow Quakers." Among the "admonitions" she had ignored were those against participating in the war. She was able to settle these conflicts during the meeting, though, and when she died in December 1789 she was buried in the Friends' cemetery not far from her home.

3

Mary Slocumb

I T WAS A BRIGHT MORNING in the spring of 1781. A British colonel on horseback dashed down the wide drive of a plantation mansion. Just behind him came his two aides, and following them were twenty mounted guards. Waiting on the road somewhat farther back were 1,100 men under the colonel's command.

Watching him rush toward her from the porch of the mansion was a very beautiful young woman. She sat with her small child, her sister, and some of the servants of the house.

The colonel drew his horse up before the porch, dismounted, and sprinted up the steps to the small group that was watching him. Ignoring the others, he made a low bow to the young woman and introduced himself as Colonel Banastre Tarleton of the British army. He knew that the young woman before him was Mary Slocumb, Patriot and wife of Lieutenant Ezekiel Slocumb of the North Carolina Patriot forces.

Tarleton commanded a part of General Cornwallis's forces that were heading north from Wilmington on their way to conquer Virginia. He could not know then that the army of 7,000 men was marching toward a surrender at the Yorktown peninsula, but just then he was not thinking of battle. He had come to announce to the young woman that he had chosen her plantation as a bivouac for his troops.

Tarleton asked Mary about her husband. She told him that he was not at home. He asked her if her husband was a rebel, to which she replied that he was fighting the invaders of his country, and therefore was not a rebel. Tarleton parried; he offered that if her husband was a friend of his country he would be a friend of their master, the king. Mary gave him no respite. In this country, she told him, only slaves looked to masters.

Mary's arrow hit home. Tarleton turned red, and ordered his aides to pitch camp.

Tarleton had underestimated Mary's nerve. She was only twenty-one, but she had been managing the plantation for five years. In this time she had learned to deal with both the plantation and the Loyalists.

She had been born in 1760 in Bertie County on Albemarle Sound in eastern North Carolina. When she was just a young child, her mother died. In 1775 her father remarried, and at his wedding Mary met her new stepbrother for the first time. They fell in love immediately, and in less than a year they were married. He took her to his plantation on the Neuse River in Wayne County in North Carolina, about eighty miles inland from the coast.

The Revolution had begun in that colony more than a year before independence was declared in Philadelphia. In May 1775 a group of citizens met in Charlotte, in Mecklenburg County in the western part of the colony. In the Mecklenburg Resolutions, published at the end of the month, they rejected the rule of king and Parliament and called for leadership from the Continental Congress.

Governor Martin was a Loyalist. In hope of suppressing the rebellion and keeping North Carolina under British rule, he issued a call for all loyal British colonists to assemble at Wilmington. He would organize them as a militia to fight the Patriots.

North Carolina had a large population of Scots. Though in their homeland the Scots constantly bristled at English rule, in America they rallied to the support of King George. Sixteen hundred Scots gathered under the command of Donald McDonald and marched off toward Wilmington and the Union Jack.

The Patriots too were assembling their forces. Led by Colonel James Moore, they aimed to ruin the Loyalists' plans to conquer the colony. Moore's strategy was to keep McDonald from reaching Wilmington. Dividing his forces, he secured important points in the area west of Wilmington through which McDonald would have to march.

Moore himself marched to Elizabethtown, on the Cape Fear River about fifty miles northwest of Wilmington. He sent Colonel Richard Casswell to take Corbett's Ferry on the Black River, and Colonels Alexander Lillington and James Ashe to rendezvous with Casswell. Zeke Slocumb and his company marched in Lillington's regiment.

Together with Casswell, Lillington and Ashe marched toward Moore's Creek Bridge, about eighteen miles from Wilmington. This bridge was the most important of all the targets, for it was on the main road to Wilmington and McDonald would have to cross it.

On the night of February 26, McDonald's men were struggling through swamps and brush on their march toward the bridge. The Patriots, now numbering 1,100, reached the bridge that night and prepared a trap. They pulled up the board flooring of the bridge, leaving only the hewn beams on which to make a crossing. In order to make the crossing nearly impossible, they smeared the beams with tallow and soap. Then they withdrew into the bushes to await the Scots.

While Casswell was preparing his trap, Mary was in her bedroom having a nightmare. She had seen her husband off from the plantation on Sunday morning, leading his company of eighty men, volunteers from the Neuse region. In her own words, "they got off in high spirits, every man stepping high and light," and full of "mischief."

All day Monday as she had worked at the mansion, she was obsessed with worries about her husband and his men. She wondered how far they had marched, where the Loyalists were, and whether Zeke was safe. Monday night as she slept restlessly, she dreamed of a battle and saw among the dead and dying a body wrapped in a bloody military cloak. The cloak was her husband's. She screamed and leaped from her bed and rushed to her husband's body; she awoke when she crashed into the wall of her room.

She found her room quiet; the fire was glowing and her child was peacefully sleeping, but her woman servant had been alarmed by the scream and the crash.

Mary thought over her experience for a short time, then announced to her servant, "I must go to him." She dressed for riding, told her anxious servant to watch the child and lock the house, and went to the stable to saddle her fast mare. She set off at a gallop down the road her husband had marched a day and a half earlier.

Mary was at first seized with doubt, but the farther she rode the more confident she became. She kept following the route she knew her husband had taken, though she did not know exactly where she would meet him. She was convinced she would find him either dead or dying.

She rode all night toward Wilmington, while her husband helped ready the trap toward which McDonald marched.

By dawn on Tuesday she had covered thirty miles. She came upon a group of women and children in the road who were anxious and fearful; they too wanted to know what was happening. From them Mary found out that Casswell's forces had split off the main road toward a town called North West, about a dozen miles from Wilmington. This route would take them across Moore's Creek Bridge. Mary set off again, following a trail left by the troops across a long stretch of barren and swampy ground.

At about eight or nine o'clock, she heard the sound of thunder and drew up her mare. Although she had never heard it before, she knew it was made by cannon. She realized that she had come to the battle of her nightmare, and for a moment she felt foolish. All night she had been convinced that her husband was already dead, but the battle was taking place only now.

Since she was nearly on top of the battle, she decided to go ahead to it and see how her husband and his men fared. She rode on further, and soon she knew the battle was very near by the sounds of muskets and rifles and the shouting of troops.

Mary galloped her mare down the trail toward the noise and in a moment was on the Wilmington road just a few hundred yards from Moore's Creek Bridge. She had ridden directly into the scene of her nightmare. Under a cluster of trees along the road were the wounded and dying men, exactly as she had seen them the night before. She scanned the scene in amazement until she found something that made her jump from her mare and run. On the ground was a body wrapped in her husband's cloak. Opening the bloody wrap, she saw "a face clothed with gore from a dreadful wound across the temple." She put her hand on the man's face—he was still warm, and when her hand touched him, he begged for a drink of water. But she did not recognize his voice.

There was no water at hand, but she found a kettle on the ground with which she got some water from a stream and brought it to the wounded man. She poured some in his mouth and rinsed his face; it was not her husband but Frank Codgell, a man she knew. He began to revive, and he told her it was not the wound in his head that was killing him but the hole in his leg. Mary looked down and saw a pool of blood at his feet. With his knife she cut away the leg of his trousers and stocking and found a bullet hole clear through his calf.

She had no bandages with her, and she could find nothing else to use but some large leaves. These she plastered to the hole and soon the bleeding stopped. There were about twenty other men under the trees, and when she had made Codgell more comfortable, she went to help them as well.

While she was about her nursing, Casswell himself appeared, amazed to see her. She was too busy to explain her presence to him, so she told him simply that she thought they would need a nurse and scolded Casswell for not having someone take care of the wounded men. As she was giving Codgell more water, her husband came upon the scene, "as bloody as a butcher and muddy as a ditcher."

Zeke was tired but contented after the battle, and Mary's presence was a happy surprise.

"Why, Mary! What are you doing there? Hugging Frank Codgell, the greatest reprobate in the army?"

"I don't care! Frank is a brave fellow, a good soldier, and a true friend to Congress!"

Casswell himself, affected by the vehemence of her answer, said, "True, true! Every word of it! You are right, madam!" And he made a low bow to her.

Mary stayed at the scene all day and far into the night. She did not tell her husband the story of her dream; she was overjoyed to see him unhurt, and he was happy that she had come.

The Patriots had scored a tremendous and decisive victory in the battle. McDonald had come to the bridge with 1,600 men and had marched them right into the trap Casswell had set. As they tried to get across the slippery beams, the Patriots opened fire on them. For three minutes Casswell's troops poured bullets on the Scots before they fled, leaving one of their commanders dead and fifty others dead or wounded. Zeke Slocumb and the other Patriots chased the survivors and captured a large number of prisoners. The Patriots suffered only one fatality.

Moore arrived soon after a battle with another company of troops, and he too went after the fleeing Loyalists. He captured a great deal of war material: 350 guns, 1,500 rifles, 150 swords and daggers, 13 wagons, and £1500 in gold from their war chest. He also captured a number of Loyalist officers, including McDonald himself.

The prisoners were brought to the Patriot encampment. Those who had resisted the most viciously were not taken prisoner, but killed. Mary felt sorry for the prisoners and begged Casswell to spare their lives. He promised her that he would punish only those who had murdered Patriots or burned their houses. Thus Mary saved a good number of Loyalists from execution.

Zeke wanted Mary to stay the whole night with him and ride back to the plantation the next day with a guard of troops. But Mary was too anxious to see her child and claimed that no mounted troops could keep up with her on her mare; therefore, in the middle of the night she left for the plantation. When she arrived home in the morning, her child ran to her and she took him in her arms. She had ridden over 120 miles in less than forty hours.

The Battle of Moore's Creek Bridge has since come to be called the Lexington and Concord of the South. The battle was extremely important for its consequences, for when Clinton and Cornwallis heard what had happened to McDonald they decided not to land their expeditionary forces. The colony was saved from British occupation for three years.

The war continued at the local level, though. There were constant skirmishes along the Neuse, and Zeke was often away from the plantation, patroling the countryside with his men or searching for Loyalist forces.

The British had a difficult time of it in the South, but by 1780 they had managed to secure both Georgia and South Carolina. North Carolina remained unconquered, however, and toward the end of 1780 the British moved north to try again to subdue the state.

In October of that year, a major battle occurred at King's Mountain in South Carolina, near the North Carolina border. Patriot militia from both states literally slaughtered a thousand Loyalists despite their attempts to surrender. Nathaniel Greene, a major in the Continental army, had taken over the southern American army from a less able commander and transformed it into a powerful fighting force.

In January of 1781 the British were defeated again in South Carolina at a place called the Cowpens near the North Carolina border. Patriot General Daniel Morgan lost twelve of his men, and sixty-one were wounded. Of the 1,000 British troops in the battle, Morgan and his men killed, wounded, or captured 900. Their commander, Colonel Banastre "Bloody" Tarleton, survived.

A few months later, on March 15, Cornwallis himself battled Greene's Continentals at Guilford Courthouse in north central North Carolina. Technically Cornwallis won, since he forced

Greene's men to retreat. But he did so at the price of enormous losses. This British "victory" cost so many troops that a member of Parliament complained, "Another such victory would destroy the British army!"

After this Cornwallis returned to Wilmington to resupply and reconsider his plans for North Carolina. Without waiting for instructions from London, he decided to leave North Carolina alone for a while and conquer Virginia instead, and in May 1781 he marched out of Wilmington. His route took his forces across the Neuse River. Tarleton took his regiment across near the Slocumb plantation and chose it as his bivouac.

After losing his battle of wits with Mary, Tarleton ordered his troops to pitch camp. The mansion faced east, and from it to the road a half mile away was a straight driveway about 150 feet wide. The drive was lined on both sides; on the northern edge was a rail fence eight feet high, and on the southern, a high fence and a line of trees. On the other side of this line was a large orchard of peach trees.

Tarleton wisely chose the peach orchard for his troops' encampment. There, behind the fence and the trees, his troops were well hidden from the sight of any Patriots who might come across the open field to the north. Tarleton informed Mary that, if it was not too great an inconvenience to her, he would take up quarters in her house.

Mary could accomplish nothing with further argument. She told Tarleton that she and her family were his prisoners and began preparing dinner for the household and the officers.

She could only hope that her husband would not blindly return home to be taken by Tarleton. Worse still, he might encounter the patrol that Tarleton had sent out to scout the area for Patriot forces.

She needed to get warning to him somehow. With the excuse of needing cornmeal, she sent a slave with a bag of corn to a mill a few miles away. The mill was along the road which her husband would use on his return from patrol; the slave was to wait for him to appear and warn him.

With one party hoping for Slocumb's capture and the other praying for his safety, Tarleton and his officers sat down to dinner with Mary and her family. The dinner was formal and sumptuous, consisting of boiled ham, turkey, sweet potatoes, vegetables, boiled beef, sausages, fowl, and wine.

A glass of peach brandy at the end of the meal prompted another exchange of verbal shots between Mary and Tarleton. The officers remarked on the excellence of the brandy. Upon learning that it had been made from the fruit of the orchard in which their troops were camped, they began speculating on the estates with which they would be rewarded for winning the war. Mary held her own throughout the discussion, puncturing the Loyalist dreams at every chance. The polite battle finished with her rebutting Tarleton again. No duke or king or any other royalty, she told him, would ever occupy their plantation.

Before the verbal war could resume on another issue, the sound of real bullets and guns signaled that Tarleton's patrol had encountered Zeke Slocumb. Tarleton ordered his officers to ready the troops for action, while Mary prayed that her husband had been warned in time. The slave she had sent to give him the warning, however, had not gotten very far. Excited by the spectacle of the officers and troops, he had tarried along the driveway, watching the men through the trees.

Tarleton and Mary stood on the porch listening to the gunfire as the troops were lined up to march out, and he asked her if Washington's forces were in the neighborhood. She replied that of course he must know that General Greene and the Marquis de Lafayette were in the state, and that he should not be surprised by a visit from Washington. This was not quite a lie. In fact the only troops nearby were composed of Zeke Slocumb and his few men, but Mary wanted Tarleton to think that the gunfire signaled the start of an attack by a large American force.

He ordered his troops to get ready to march out for battle, then he mounted his horse and galloped to the head of the regiment to lead it out. Mary stayed on the porch, with Tarleton's guards standing at attention in front of the house, knowing that her husband's small band would have no chance against more than a thousand soldiers. As she looked out over the fields, she suddenly gasped at a fantastic sight.

Heading south across the open ground toward the driveway came a small group of horsemen flashing swords and firing pistols. As they drew closer, Mary saw that it was a small number of Tarleton's men being chased by her husband, her brother, and the few others of their band. In the lead was the captain of the British patrol with a thirteen-year-old boy after him.

Her husband's men could not see the British regiment behind the tree line, and she watched helplessly as they chased the Loyalists directly toward it. When they reached the middle of the drive, one of the Loyalists was struck down, and in the next moment the slave who had tarried ran from the trees to shout a warning to Zeke. Slocumb drew up his horse and looked around—at the entrance to the driveway a platoon of Tarleton's cavalry was leaping the fence already. Slocumb's band wheeled around and at full gallop headed straight down the drive toward the house and the astonished guards. With Tarleton's platoon in hot pursuit they turned in front of the house, leaped the fences of the garden, then over a canal, across an open field, and, in a rain of bullets from the guards, toward a wood.

They escaped. Tarleton called back his platoon before it could cross the canal; he still thought that a large Patriot force was in the countryside around the plantation. Mary's insinuations had saved the lives of her husband and his band.

For Tarleton, the day's action was over, and he would not get another chance at Zeke Slocumb. He had lost his advantage of surprise, and he was now in more danger of being attacked than ever. He was on his way to conquer Virginia, and he did not want to be delayed for another battle in North Carolina.

Tarleton ordered his troops to return to camp and walked back to the house. He remarked to Mary that her husband had made only a short visit, and he would have liked to make his acquaintance. Mary assured him that he would sooner or later and when he did, her husband would thank him for the way he had treated his wife.

Tarleton was embarrassed. He apologized for occupying her property and explained that he did so only out of military necessity. He soon removed his troops, and as a token of his respect for her, he posted a guard at her door until the last soldier had left.

He resumed his march toward Yorktown and the British defeat in the American Revolution.

4

Margaret Corbin

THE VIOLENCE and drama of Margaret Corbin's life began almost in her infancy. She was born in November 1751 in what is now Franklin County, Pennsylvania. When she was only five years old—hardly old enough to remember her parents—her home was raided by Indians. Her father was killed, and her mother was taken away as a captive.

In these raids the Indians usually killed everyone, looted the houses, and burned whatever buildings they could. Often, however, they took young children to raise as Indians and women to become squaws or servants to squaws. Margaret's mother was one of these; she never again returned to her home, but two years later, in 1758, she was seen with the Indians in the frontier territory a hundred miles west of the Ohio River. Nothing more was ever seen or heard of her.

Margaret and her brother survived the Indian attack, but they were now parentless; a brother of Margaret's mother took them in and raised them. At age twenty-one Margaret married John Corbin who had moved to Pennsylvania from Virginia.

The Revolution broke out four years after they were married, and John immediately enlisted. He became a private in Captain Thomas Proctor's First Company of the Pennsylvania Artillery, and Margaret went with him.

The Continental army followed the custom of the British army in permitting a number of soldiers' wives to stay with each company. These women served the company as a whole; they did the cooking, the washing, the clothes-mending, and frequently nursed the sick and wounded. Such was Margaret's life with her husband in the artillery company. She was not only exposed to the dangers of war

26

as he was, but she had an enormous amount of work as well.

In Margaret's case, there was action in combat, too. After the capture of New York City by General Howe, General Washington moved north of Manhattan and held off the British for a few weeks in the Battle of Harlem Heights during September 1776. On November 16, the Hessian troops then attacked Fort Washington where Margaret and her husband were stationed. The Continentals fought to hold the fort against the large force of attackers, pitting 2,800 men against the almost 9,000 in the attacking force. Margaret's husband was killed at his cannon. There was no one else to fire it, so Margaret ran to the cannon and began loading and firing it herself. She continued firing until she herself was seriously wounded by British grapeshot.

The battle was too unequal a contest for the fort's defenders. Watching it from the Palisades at Fort Lee, Washington wept as he saw his brave soldiers being overwhelmed by the British forces. The British captured Fort Washington, and the survivors became their prisoners.

How she found her way out of British hands we do not know, but eventually Margaret made her way back to the American army. She had a very hard time of it, for her husband was dead and her wound disabled her. This disability was to stay with her the rest of her life.

It was difficult enough for a woman to survive by herself, without means and without a home, during the Revolution. But Margaret was also badly handicapped and needed others to care for her. She was now in the situation of many Revolutionary soldiers whose wounds kept them from going into combat again, and for their sake the Continental army established the Invalid Regiment in 1777. The soldiers in the Regiment were based at West Point and served as recruiters and instructors for the army.

Margaret's own state of Pennsylvania recognized her heroism and also her poverty, and in 1779 the state voted to pay her thirty dollars relief and recommended that the Board of War aid her as well. The Continental Congress allowed her a soldier's pension at one-half the rate of an active soldier's pay and an annual outfit of clothing. To receive this assistance, she enrolled in the Invalid Regiment and moved to West Point. She was the only woman in the regiment and also the first woman pensioner in the United States.

By 1782 Margaret married again, but with this move she did not solve her problem of poverty—her new husband was also an invalid and actually added to her cares. She continued to try to improve her lot though, and she petitioned for a full soldier's ration rather than only the half she was receiving. Her request was not granted, but she was allowed a full ration of rum or whiskey. (Up to this time the army had forbidden its women to use liquor.) In addition, recognizing a debt to her, the army granted her the money value of the spirits she had been denied in the previous years. With this her life became a little easier, although she still was not in comfortable circumstances.

At the close of the Revolutionary War in 1783, the Invalid Regiment was disbanded, and Margaret lived for the next several years around West Point where the military commissary provided her with the necessities of life. Later she moved to the nearby town of Highland Falls where she spent her last years.

The local people in Highland Falls knew Margaret as "Captain Molly"; she was disagreeable, bad tempered, and eccentric. Considering her difficult life, we can hardly blame these on her as faults. She usually dressed in petticoats and an artilleryman's coat. The local people respected her, and even though some who disliked her called her "Dirty Kate" behind her back, they saluted her to her face.

Margaret Corbin died in Highland Falls around 1800, and she was buried in the local cemetery. Later her remains were transferred to the cemetery at West Point, where she now lies with her comrades-in-arms of our nation's wars.

PART II

Literary Ladies

5

Esther De Berdt Reed

ESTHER DE BERDT REED was an Englishwoman who became an American Patriot during the rebellion against British rule. Migrating to America after her marriage, Esther Reed's sympathies were slowly weaned from her motherland by the mismanagement of colonial relations in the period preceding the Revolutionary War. After she was convinced of the necessity for armed resistance, she was no lukewarm Patriot with shifting and ambiguous commitment; rather, she was identified by her community as a convinced revolutionary. Her beliefs are clearly expressed in the many letters written to her fiancé, Joseph Reed, and later to her English brother, Dennis De Berdt. These letters still serve to enlighten us about the Revolutionary War era as experienced on both sides of the Atlantic. But Esther Reed did not merely scribble her ideas on a piece of paper; she put them into practice.

While recovering from smallpox, she personally led a vigorous campaign to wrest the last hoarded shilling from the households of both Philadelphia and Germantown to support the soldiers in George Washington's army. By July 4, 1780, Esther Reed and her committee had gathered thousands of Continental dollars. Even while she was arranging the form of distribution and working to establish local committees in other towns, she contracted dysentery and died.

In adolescence Esther Reed had developed a stern capacity for self-sacrifice. Her father, Dennys De Berdt, was a wealthy British merchant in the colonial trade. His dealings with the colonies led to his being chosen agent for both Delaware and Massachusetts during the Stamp Act crisis of the mid-1760s. As a young woman of twenty, Esther observed with keen appreciation her father's negotiations with members of both houses of Parliament. While Dennys De Berdt attempted to secure repeal of a bill which was disadvantageous to the colonies and his own enterprise, his daughter was required to negotiate even more delicate situations to maintain the family's social standing despite their political unpopularity.

At a time when her father's politics were making social relations sticky, Esther De Berdt turned toward the frequent houseguests from America for diversion. The De Berdt household was a gathering place for young Americans who were in England to be educated in business and law. It was also the political center in which colonial agents gathered to hammer out unified positions in keeping with their instructions from colonial legislatures. Only Benjamin Franklin exempted himself from these strategy sessions, having his own connections with Parliament.

When these Americans met their young hostess in De Berdt's London home or country house at Enfield, many were impressed by her. Of a lithe, almost ethereal frame, Esther De Berdt was a studious and profoundly religious young woman. It is not surprising that several of De Berdt's visitors courted his daughter. Those who did so soon discovered that the delicacy of her appearance concealed a quick mind and an animated spirit. There was one young American who won the attention and soon the affections of Esther De Berdt. Joseph Reed was a student of law whose personal career was advanced by his association with Dennys De Berdt.

In the De Berdt houses in London and Enfield, Joseph Reed pressed his suit, much to the consternation of Esther's parents. For the well-established De Berdt family, a young American lawyer of no great repute or family connections was not a suitable match, however attractive and intelligent he might be. They preferred a young aristocrat or successful merchant of a good English family. The most unsuitable aspect of this proposed match was that Esther might be removed from England to America. Englishmen of De Berdt's class were convinced that America was still an inhospitable desert.

The De Berdt family finally consented to a correspondence between the couple while Joseph returned to his country. When he sailed for America on February 7, 1765, it was his hope to transfer his business and legal affairs to London as soon as possible, but the colonies were separated from the British Isles by a wide and dangerous sea passage and by an increasingly dangerous political gulf. Parliament passed the Stamp Act on March 22, 1765, before Reed's ship reached America.

Parliament passed this bill at the behest of the Grenville ministry which hoped to defray the costs of running the empire and to repay war debts accumulated in the costly imperial wars of the first part of the eighteenth century. Americans reacted angrily. This was the first tax, other than customs duties, to be enacted in Parliament for the colonies. Many were concerned lest the requirement for payment in specie would further contract the colonial money supply. This act represented an important change of situation for the colonies, since their merchants could not expect the British Parliament to permit prosperity in America as long as Britain had debts. Though the tax itself was not high, Americans feared it would provide a dangerous precedent. Virtually every piece of paper of any legal or social significance was taxed, including a £10 tax on Joseph Reed's legal license and a shilling tax on his pack of playing cards.

When Joseph arrived in America, he found that his family's situation had worsened during his absence. His father was aging and ill. His brother had been profligate with family resources and had abandoned his responsibilities. At a time when he had hoped to conclude his American affairs to claim his British bride, Joseph Reed had the support of a large American family thrust upon him. For five lonely years Joseph and Esther corresponded across an ocean which frequently swallowed their letters.

A very accurate picture of the development of British and American political opinions can be drawn from the correspondence between Esther De Berdt and Joseph Reed during the period 1765-1770. One reason for their early preoccupation with politics was their hope that Joseph could return to help Dennys De Berdt if the elder man was made permanent agent of Massachusetts with a large salary. Even though politics fascinated this young couple, they deplored its effect on their own lives. In August 1767, Joseph wrote to Esther about the feuds in the Boston Assembly: "I have often lamented that our happiness depended on the unsteady flame of politics, but never felt the disappointment and chagrin arising from it more keenly than I did this morning when I received Sayre's letter, informing me that the Governor and Council had not confirmed your father's appointment."

Esther's perceptions about the political future of the empire were usually accurate. In August 1768 Esther wrote to Joseph of her anxiety about relations between America and England: "There is a storm gathering, which will break over England as well as America, and what will be the consequence it is impossible to say." Engaged secretly to an American, Esther found occasion to remark on the growth of popular contempt for Americans as resistance began in the colonies. "To be an American or a friend of America, is a great disadvantage," wrote Esther in January 1769. In a letter written the next month, she suggested that the bad feeling between England and America might be irreversible. "In this melancholy situation of things, it is impossible for anyone to stem the tide against America."

The tide *was* running against America. Parliament asserted its claim to authority over taxation. A repressive policy was instituted to permit trial of American cases in Admiralty courts far from the location of the alleged offense. At this time of high feeling against America, Joseph Reed determined to return to England and claim his bride. He had given up the plan to transfer his affairs to that country, but he hoped to bring Esther back to America. If she could not leave England, Joseph Reed was resolved to settle there without any sure means of support.

Joseph Reed arrived in England during the first week of May 1770, after five years' absence from his intended bride. He discovered that Dennys De Berdt had just died, leaving his business in disorder. His beloved Esther met him with sorrow rather than the joy he had hoped to find. Several days after his arrival he described the situation to his brother-in-law, Mr. Pettit:

> I found my worthy friend gone, my dear girl almost worn out with sorrow and fatigue, and the whole family in a situation not to be described. . . . It is indeed a melancholy scene to look through the books of this house, which show a very handsome fortune acquired, and, I fear, lost again, by credulity on the part of Mr. De Berdt and dishonesty on the part of many of our countrymen. . . . Mrs. De Berdt and her daughter have consented to go to America if it appears necessary, but I doubt that the former would be happy there. A change at her time of life would be disagreeable.

Had any of the De Berdt family thought Joseph's interest in Esther was stimulated by her station in the society of wealthy British merchants, his fidelity at this time of family ruin must have proved otherwise. Joseph and Esther were married at St. Luke's Church in London on May 22, 1770, just seven weeks after her father's death. The Reeds sailed with Mrs. De Berdt to America.

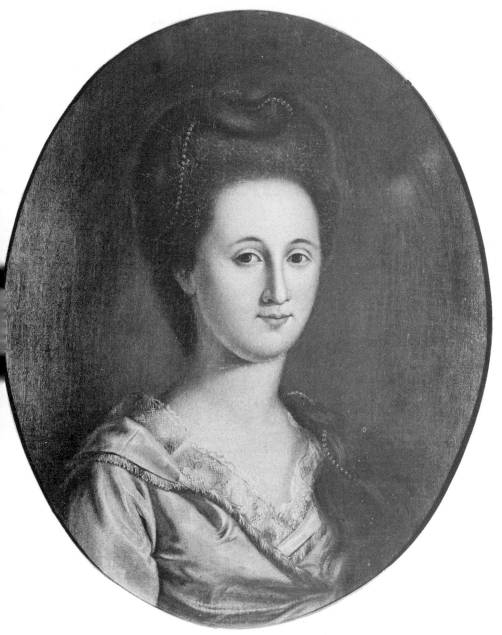

Esther De Berdt Reed (Portrait by C. W. Peale)
Courtesy, Frick Art Reference Library

Esther's life following her arrival in America was very happy. She was pleased with the husband she had longed for during Joseph's five-year absence, and she clung with even more devotion to him because she was among unfamiliar people in a strange land. Joseph Reed became a leading Patriot and Esther identified herself with her husband's cause, though she longed to return to England.

Much is known about the gradual shift in Esther De Berdt Reed's loyalties because her letters to her brother in England were quite open and extensive. Politics was mingled with news of their mother and Esther's new family. Almost a year after her marriage, when her first daughter was born, Esther wrote that she was content with life in the colonies only for the present. Rather than reconciling her to America, the birth of Esther's daughter had made the return to England seem more imperative. "If she lives, it will make me more anxious than ever to return to dear England, as the education of girls is very indifferent indeed here." She was dissatisfied with the level of education and intellectual accomplishment attained by her Philadelphia acquaintances.

After more than two years of marriage and life in America, Esther found it more attractive but still she longed to return to England. She was not yet American at heart when she wrote to her brother Dennis in October 1772:

> I think that I never enjoyed a greater share of health and spirits; nothing is wanting but clearer prospects of returning to dear England; it would indeed rejoice my heart, once more to set my foot on that charming island. America must be allowed to be a fine country, but the conveniences and elegancies of England are unrivaled; they are not to be expected here; but I make myself contented.

Until her fourth year of marriage Esther continued to hope for a return to England, as her husband became an increasingly important spokesman for the Patriot movement.

In the fall of 1774, Esther Reed entertained in her home many members of the First Continental Congress, then meeting in Philadelphia. Among her guests were George Washington and John and Samuel Adams. She was glowingly described by a Connecticut member on this occasion as a "daughter of Liberty, zealously affected in a good Cause." Esther De Berdt Reed had once again concerned herself with the intricacies of politics. She felt that America had been wronged by Parliament.

To enforce the tea tax and to punish Massachusetts for disobedience and protest, Parliament passed a series of Coercive Acts in the spring of 1774. The first of these acts was an order to close the port of Boston to trade for an indefinite time, if not forever. This act was aimed directly at the Bostonians who had sanctioned such destruction of property as the Boston Tea Party. If the act had been enforced, the city with which Dennys De Berdt had done much of his trade would have been finished as a commercial center. Since the council had been unwilling to support the governor openly during the crisis, a second act provided for royal appointment of council members.

The acts directed against Boston and Massachusetts were designed to have an instructive effect in the other colonies. Parliament also undertook to provide legal protection for soldiers during future incidents like the Boston Massacre. The Administration of Justice Act was passed to protect royal officers who might be accused of capital crimes in the performance of their duties anywhere in the colonies. This and the Quartering Act, which provided for the maintenance of a standing army in their midst, convinced many colonists that the British were determined to force colonial submission to the will of Parliament even at the cost of bloodshed.

Esther wrote urgently to her brother Dennis of her horror at the prospect of war in the colonies. At this point she spoke as an American, anguished that her homeland might be torn and ravaged by a terrible war:

> The next news from England after Parliament meets, I imagine, will be decisive. May God grant it may not be hostile. A determination to proceed and inforce [*sic*] must inevitably plunge New England into a scene of blood and all the horrors of civil war, and how far it would extend it is impossible to say.

Esther was not so affected by her vision of terror that she was unable to weigh carefully the political predictions she had heard around her. "Many people here," she reported, "are very sanguine in their expectations that the Acts will be repealed immediately . . . but I cannot believe any such happy change will speedily take place. The people of New England have not such expectations." (November 1774)

Esther indicated in her letter to Dennis that her expectation that the situation would not easily be defused was shared by the people of New England. She went on to discuss the position held by the New Englanders whom she had met:

> They are prepared for the worst event, and they have such ideas of
> their injured liberty, and so much enthusiasm for the cause, that I do
> not think that any power on earth could take it from them but with
> their lives.

Finally, Esther assured her brother that further reprisals against
Massachusetts would not isolate it from the other colonies. She also
cautioned him against thinking that the Continental Congress was a
radical group out of sympathy with the general opinions of the
colonists.

> The proceedings of Congress will show you how united the whole
> continent is in the cause and from them you may judge of the sense
> of the people.

Esther revealed an ungrudging admiration for the zeal of Massachusetts. She never expressed hope that the people of New England
would recognize the legitimacy of Parliamentary rule within the
colony. The ideas expressed in her letters to Dennis showed that
Esther De Berdt Reed had begun to identify herself as an American
and as a Patriot.

Though she hoped in her November letter that moderation could
prevent bloodshed, by February 1775 Esther felt that the movement
toward war might be inexorable. Fearing that it might ruin the
country, she was cheered nonetheless by the general agreement
among the people of its necessity. The terrors of war were clearly on
the horizon when she wrote to Dennis:

> One great comfort I have is, that if these great affairs must be brought
> to a crisis and decided, it had better be in our time than in our
> children's.

Esther De Berdt Reed felt that the issues at stake were well worth
fighting for if they could not otherwise be resolved. She did not
mention any wish to escape the coming war by fleeing to the
homeland she had left five years earlier.

By June 1775 Joseph Reed had been appointed lieutenant colonel
of the Philadelphia battalion of the Pennsylvania militia. Having
cast his lot with the revolution, Joseph probably no longer intended
to return to England. Esther admitted in correspondence with
Dennis that return to England was presently impossible. In July

Joseph Reed was appointed temporary secretary to General Washington, then at Cambridge.

During the war years, Esther Reed's letters served as a means of communication with the British mercantile class, to which her brother belonged. She articulated the ideals of the revolution and memorialized its accomplishments. Her first wartime letter was written soon after her husband had been called north to join Washington's army. She described the total involvement of the populace in wartime effort and sacrifice.

> The whole continent is so engaged now that they will never give up. Georgia has joined the Congress—every heart and hand almost, is warm and active in the cause: certainly, my dear brother, it is a glorious one. You see every person willing to sacrifice his private interest in this glorious contest. Virtue, honour, unanimity, bravery,—all conspire to carry it on, and sure it has at least a chance to be victorious.

After asserting the strength of public commitment to the cause, Esther felt justified in her own belief in the final certainty of victory. To those who had known her as a gentle Englishwoman only five years earlier, this passion for the American cause must have been striking.

In September Esther wrote to Dennis that she was relieved that her husband's life was not then endangered, though his business profits had been sacrificed. Despite the burden of small children, inflation, and the uncertainty of war, Esther accepted her husband's absence. As the American forces suffered setbacks, her anger at the British pursuit of victory grew.

> But where sleep all our friends in England? Where sleep the virtue and justice of the English nation? Will nothing arouse them, or are they so few in number and small in consequence that though awake, their voice cannot be heard for the multitude of our enemies.

She reflected that she might not have left England had she known the future of the colonies. She did not regret being in the conflict because "our country would not have been benefited, for at this time she requires all her friends, and has a right to expect services from such heads and hearts, as can most conduce to her safety."

In correspondence with Dennis De Berdt, Esther Reed was

among the first colonists to suggest to Englishmen that American independence was inevitable if reconciliation was not soon undertaken. In a letter of October 28, 1775, Esther's discussion of trade possibilities with the empire led to the subject of American independence. Dennis was hoping to establish his fortune in trade with America.

> As to trade, it hangs so uncertain, that we may in a few months trade with all the world on our own risk, or it may return to its former Channel. It seems now to depend on the reception of our last Petition from the Congress to the King; if that would be so considered as to lay a foundation for negotiation, we may be again reconciled,—if not, I imagine WE SHALL DECLARE FOR INDEPENDENCE, and exert our utmost to defend ourselves.

The connection between trade and independence was as intimate as Esther described it in her letter to Dennis. Resistance could not be successful without foreign aid, which could only be obtained with the offer of free access to American trade after the victory.

Esther Reed was aware of how quickly her affections had become allied to America's cause. She knew that in the fall of 1775 she held ideas which would have seemed treasonous to her only a few years earlier.

> This proposition for independence would have alarmed almost every person on the Continent a twelve-month ago, but now the general voice is, if the Ministry and the Nation will drive us to it, we must do it, rather than submit, after so many public resolutions to the contrary.

The war years were physically punishing for Esther Reed. She was left alone in charge of a family growing from three children to six, and her husband was subject to danger and misfortune as an aide to General Washington. Despite her suffering, Esther's letters to her husband were always supportive of his participation in the military effort. This is shown in one missive written in June 1777 while Joseph was with the American army at its headquarters in Middlebrook, New Jersey. Esther was with her family at Norristown, Pennsylvania, about seventeen miles from Philadelphia.

> I wish I could find words sufficient to express how much I approve and admire your conduct, in which the tenderest regard for my

happiness mingles with your disinterested exertions in your country's
service, but I dare not say all I think,—I know you smile already at
what you call my partiality,—but I know my dear friend will not
wholly despise my praises.

Though she and Joseph had known and loved each other for
twelve years, only five had been spent in the same home together.

Joseph Reed described his wife's wartime burden in a letter
written in May 1778 to Esther's English brother. He reported the
loss of two-year-old Theodosia by smallpox and told of the birth of a
son. Though Joseph minimized the family's material losses in the
war, he wrote, "We have been obliged to move four times and had
our house once plundered away by the enemy."

Joseph Reed's military service during the Revolutionary War was
competent though not really distinguished. After serving as Washington's secretary, he was appointed adjutant general. In that
position he trained a continuous supply of new troops and attempted to equip them from the summer of 1776 to the spring of 1777. He
resigned as adjutant general to be appointed to the command of the
cavalry, which he hoped would be enlarged to 3,000. Political
infighting over the prestigious cavalry command led Joseph to
choose instead to serve as Washington's aide. With Washington,
Reed was in every important campaign. Though he was not
seriously injured, two horses were killed beneath him, and on at
least one occasion, he believed himself taken prisoner. Though
Esther had always avoided burdening her husband with her own
fears for his welfare, Joseph knew she was happy when he left active
military duty for a seat in the Congress in the winter of 1777-78. He
wrote Dennis:

> Your sister (though she has supported this, as well as everything else,
> with great firmness) is so much affected at the risk of a military life,
> that last fall I accepted a seat in Congress, to which I had long been
> solicited. . . .

In December 1778 Joseph Reed was elected president of the
Executive Council of the state of Pennsylvania, and Esther Reed
assumed new duties and pleasures. Formerly lonely during her
husband's absence, she was now one of the leading figures in the
most dazzling social life in all of the American states. Her longing
for the elegance of London twelve years earlier was fulfilled, but it
was tempered by her position. She was forced to help maintain a

delicate balance between unalterably hostile parties. She was sometimes excessive in her effort to achieve some measure of Republican austerity in wartime. Both she and her husband frowned on the glitter and luxury of Benedict Arnold's military government in Philadelphia. At least one group—the formerly powerful Loyalist women, such as the Chews and Shippens—made her the subject of satire and acidic comment. The anxieties of administering a wartorn city and state were the cause of the first strife between Joseph and Esther.

After a serious bout with smallpox, which endangered the lives of her remaining five children, Esther launched a new project which she hoped would unify people from all social classes in Philadelphia. The soldiers in General Washington's army were suffering the worst hardships of the war in 1780. The American army emerged from winter retreat in tattered coats, ragged regimentals, and advanced stages of dysentery, smallpox, and cholera. The prominent Patriot ladies of Philadelphia joined with Esther Reed in a drive to gather money to obtain additional supplies for the soldiers.

Correspondence between the Reeds and the commander in chief on the subject of shirts was begun on January 20, 1780. Joseph Reed wrote to Washington to announce that a campaign to gather money from the households of Philadelphia had been undertaken by a women's committee.

> The ladies have caught the happy contagion, and in a few days, Mrs. Reed will have the honour of writing to you on the subject. It is expected that she will have a sum equal to £100,000 [currency], to be laid out according to your Excellency's direction, in such a way as may be thought most honorable and gratifying to the brave old soldiers who have borne so great a share of the burden of this war. I thought it best to mention it in this way to your Excellency for your consideration, as it may tend to forward the benevolent scheme of the donors with dispatch. I must observe that the ladies have excepted such articles of necessity as clothing which the States are bound to provide.

Washington acknowledged the value of the donations, but he suggested that articles of linen clothing were needed most by the soldiers.

The final results of labors in Philadelphia, Germantown, rural Pennsylvania, and New Jersey was a fund consisting of many thousands of Continental dollars, gathered mostly from the housekeeping accounts of women. In her letter to Washington describing the dimensions of the collection, Esther Reed suggested that the true meaning of the fund lay in its evidence that the contributors were zealous Patriots grateful for the bravery of their army.

> . . . although it has answered our expectations, it does not equal our wishes, but I am persuaded the money will be received as a proof of our zeal for the great cause of America and our esteem and gratitude for those who so bravely defend it.

She concluded the letter with a statement of her intention to execute any design for the money that Washington might offer which was consistent with the intentions of the donors.

In his response to Esther Reed's communication, Washington once again suggested that linen clothing was what the soldiers needed most. In addition to recommending that they purchase linen and manufacture shirts for the men, Washington suggested that a fund of that size could be used to strengthen the bank. He proposed the collection be deposited in the bank and that bank notes be used to obtain the linen. Washington seemed to ignore the ladies' intention not to duplicate any provision which the states were bound to give the troops.

When she learned of the commander in chief's continued insistence that the money be invested in linen and then manufactured into shirts, Esther Reed found a supplier of linen. Before the actual manufacture of shirts was begun Esther wrote again to Washington. In her letter she pointed out that Pennsylvania had just sent 2,000 shirts in July 1780 and that the French fleet had landed a large shipment of shirts. She hoped to contrive another means of conveying the gift from the ladies of Pennsylvania. She described the use most favored by the ladies.

> . . . an idea prevails among the ladies, that the soldiers will not be so much gratified, by bestowing an article to which they are entitled from the public, as in some other method which will convey more fully the idea of a reward for past services, and an incitement to future duty. Those who are of this opinion propose the whole of the money to be changed into hard dollars, and giving each soldier two, to be entirely at his own disposal.

If the general concurred with this plan to distribute hard currency despite a continued need for linen shirts, Esther promised that the state of Pennsylvania would meet the deficiency for its own armies and would try to provide for the neglected soldiers of other states.

Unfortunately, the supply of the barest necessities was so poor that George Washington felt constrained to reiterate his request that specific supplies of clothing rather than hard cash be sent to the troops. Esther Reed wrote again expressing her acquiescence with Washington's request. The stiff formality of Washington's reply to her letter suggesting the gift of hard currency led Esther to believe that he had been piqued at being asked a second time for his opinion. It was unlikely that very many Americans of either sex asked the general to reconsider any decision. The thirty-nine women on the committee immediately began cutting and sewing shirts.

Less than two weeks after the manufacture of shirts was begun, Esther Reed became gravely ill. Already weakened by an earlier bout with smallpox, by childbirth, and by the anxieties of war, Esther's illness was brief. She died of acute dysentery on September 22, 1780, at the age of thirty-three. Her work in manufacturing shirts for the army was continued under the leadership of Sarah Franklin Bache. More than 2,000 shirts were delivered to the army by the year's end. As much a victim of the war as if she had died at Valley Forge from the same disease, the young Englishwoman who became an American Patriot left five children all under fourteen years of age.

6

Mercy Otis Warren

IN 1805 a handsomely bound three-volume set entitled *History of the Rise, Progress, and Termination of the American Revolution* was published in Boston. Begun almost thirty years before, it chronicled the sweeping events from the outset of the war to Jefferson's first administration. It was a moral history, less concerned with famous battles and heroic accomplishments than with passing judgment on the deeds of men and the philosophical issues surrounding the birth of a new nation. Idealistic and intensely argued, it attempted to explain the Revolution in terms of a reconciliation between Puritan manners and morality and the enlightened social thought of the eighteenth century. Among historians and other intellectuals both in Europe and America, it was held in high regard and survived as an important document well into the nineteenth century.

But by far the most interesting fact regarding this history is that it was written by a woman. The author, Mercy Otis Warren, was one of Massachusetts's best known writers throughout the revolutionary period. As a woman in a decidedly male-dominated intellectual world, her achievements are overwhelming. Though there have been recurrent attempts to revive this great person's reputation, it is surprising that she is not better known in our own day.

Mercy was the third of thirteen children born to the Otises of Barnstable on Cape Cod. It was an old and respected family of moderate wealth—aristocracy of a peculiarly American kind. In 1728 Barnstable was not yet a hundred years old, and the local "royalty" was composed of those known to be descended from the first colonists of the Massachusetts region. Mercy's father, Colonel James, was a fourth generation American, though it was her mother, Mary Allyne, who had the most formidable lineage. Her great-grandfather, Edward Dotey, had arrived on the *Mayflower* and, incidentally, was the first person to fight a duel in the New World. The family seems to have prospered after this rough beginning.

The colonel was a man of boundless energy—a successful merchant and farmer, a deacon of the church, and a self-taught lawyer who was admitted to the Massachusetts bar. Like his father before him, James dominated the political life of Barnstable and would soon find himself embroiled in the more elevated and treacherous politics of Boston.

Of his wife there is little record other than that she spent two decades bearing children and that she was devoutly religious and intensely domestic. Religion, in fact, was central to the life of the Otises, not merely in the church-going sense, but in their deep Puritan convictions about man's dependency on God, the virtuous life and, above all, duty—that most comprehensive and dominating word in the Puritan vocabulary.

With a mother of such strong domestic inclinations, young Mercy was naturally trained in all the household skills from an early age. Sewing, cooking, embroidery, soap-making, laced with a bit of basic reading, writing, and arithmetic—this was the standard fare of women's education in the Otises' class. Mercy found no difficulty in accepting this housewifely role, and she would not in later years. The overriding concern with duty, so thoroughly communicated by her mother, became a part of every aspect of her life. It would give her the strength to become the exceptional person she was.

Her firm character was also shaped by other influences that few young women of her time could have hoped for or would have taken advantage of. Her older brother by three years was James Otis, Jr., called Jemmy. His effect on his sister's life would be immeasurable, just as it would be on the course of the Revolution. As the split deepened between Britain and her colonies, James's activities would cause him to be known simply as "The Patriot." It was an apt title, for he was one of the key figures in laying the foundation for American independence. Through him a whole world generally denied to women would open up for Mercy.

It began at Barnstable. The pastor of the local congregation, Jonathon Russell, was a graduate of Yale renowned for his learning. He was also the brother-in-law of Colonel James Otis. The colonel wondered if Russell would like to augment his income by tutoring a

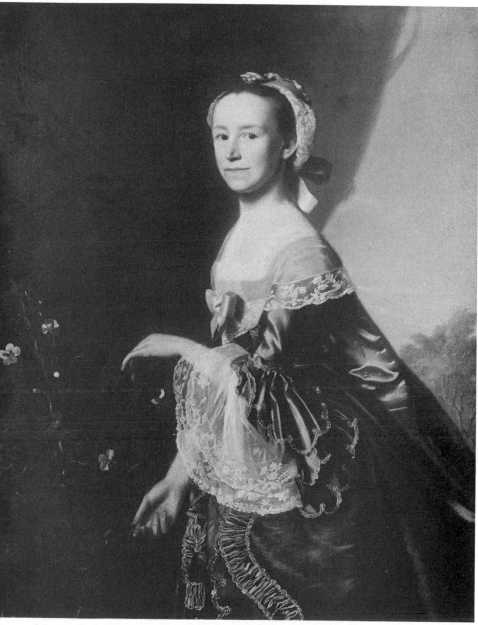

Mercy Otis Warren (Portrait by John Singleton Copley)
Courtesy, Museum of Fine Arts, Boston.

few exceptional students. Russell agreed and, not surprisingly, his first students were Jemmy and his brother Joseph.

What was truly surprising, however, is that when the Otis brothers took their seats in Mr. Russell's parish house each day, their little sister, Mercy, was with them. For the next several years she would receive the same schooling as her brothers, with the exception of formal studies in Latin and Greek.

And what did Joseph and James Jr. think of this? Jemmy took an active role in sharing his studies with his sister and tutoring her at home; as students, the two were inseparable. Joseph, on the other hand, was more of a free spirit and less inclined to Russell's discipline. He dropped out of the school early and went into the family business.

Mercy's formal education continued until she was about fifteen, long after Joseph had quit and Jemmy was installed at Harvard. It seems that she demonstrated such exceptional interest and ability at an early age that she couldn't be ignored. Perhaps the family initiated her education at first as a bit of a lark—amused that a young girl should have such proclivities—but it soon became apparent that Mercy's talents were to be taken seriously.

Unlike many of his fellow ministers, Russell's tastes went beyond religious philosophy to literature, both classical and modern. Mercy developed an intense interest in both. Ironically, while Jemmy labored through Virgil and Homer in the originals to learn the grammar that was part of classical education, Mercy was free to speed through the English translations by Pope and Dryden, along with the works of Cicero, Shakespeare, and Milton. It is certain that by the time Jemmy left for Harvard at age thirteen, his ten-year-old sister was far better read than he was. This was fairly weighty literature for children and, in part, it accounts for the lethargy that developed in many young students at the time. But Mercy seemed to flourish under the rigors of formal training and the heavy didacticism that characterized much of the literature of her time. At the same time she was developing a phenomenal memory and these early lessons became a part of her lifelong intellectual makeup.

The most important lesson she learned from Jonathon Russell influenced her ability to write. Writing was usually considered a necessity that might be developed with a bit of style, but it was looked on more as a useful tool than an end in itself. Russell, however, was of a new line of preachers who rejected the old Puritan standard that the word of God could only come through his ministers on earth in an extemporaneous manner. Russell carefully wrote out his sermons in advance, weighing his words, choosing the right phrases, and balancing clarity with elegance. Mercy was intrigued with the power of words when care was taken with them. She noted the effect of careful language in her favorite poets, Pope and Dryden. Walter Raleigh's *History of the World* had a profound effect on her, for not only was it sweeping in scope but it also combined an elegance of form with a moral view of history that matched her growing preoccupations under Russell's tutelage. At a time when most girls of her age and class learned only the florid letter-writing style of high-born women, Mercy had as her models the best in poetry, history, and philosophy. They would be clearly evident in her writing style for the rest of her life.

These early years were a great joy to Mercy, not only because of the perfect mentor she had found in Jonathon Russell, but also because she was daily in the company of Jemmy—her idol and perhaps the greatest single influence in her life. Now, however, her brother was off for four years at Harvard, and she would see him only rarely. His departure left a great void in her life, which she filled with domestic chores and more intense work in Mr. Russell's library than before.

Jemmy's scholarship reached a formidable level by the time he graduated, and as was the custom, he gave his own commencement party to which family and friends were invited. It was the first time that fifteen-year-old Mercy had been outside Barnstable. There she met James Warren, a friend and classmate of Jemmy's from Plymouth. The young Warren and the Otises both shared a common ancestor—that prolific old Puritan, Edward Dotey. At the time of their meeting, Mercy and young Warren could not have imagined what the future held for them.

For the next two years Mercy and Jemmy were united once again—Jemmy studying for his master's degree, Mercy studying along with him. Both found themselves becoming deeply involved in John Locke's *Essays on Government*, which provided them with the republican attitudes that would characterize their activities in years to come.

After receiving his master's, Jemmy went to Boston where he studied law for two years with Jeremiah Gridley, the attorney general of Massachusetts. In 1748 he opened his own law office in Plymouth, a short distance from Barnstable. Throughout this time James Warren, Jemmy's former classmate, had been a regular visitor to the Otis farm. Ostensibly he came to see his old school friend, Jemmy, but it was clear that James and Mercy had been fond of each other since that probable first meeting at Harvard. James was extraordinarily conservative in his private behavior, and the relationship was slow in developing. By 1754, however, it appears that he was ready to assume responsibility for a family and his own portion of the estate. Neither the Warrens nor the Otises could have had any objection to the match—it was an auspicious joining of two wealthy families, James and Mercy were highly regarded by each other's parents, and they were in love. In November they were married in a simple ceremony and went to live at the Warren farm on the Eel River, a few miles outside of Plymouth. He was twenty-eight; she was twenty-six.

Jemmy, by this time, had already made his mark as an attorney. He commanded huge fees and was in demand at trials as far away as Maine and Philadelphia. He was probably unmatched in legal argument and won most of his cases by the sheer weight of his logic and his eloquence in the courtroom. But something else was growing in his mind.

Back in his postgraduate days at Barnstable, Jemmy had occasionally behaved in a peculiar fashion. He would wander alone in the woods for days at a time without speaking to anyone, and then, just as suddenly, become so talkative and quarrelsome that no one could get a word in edgewise. In the midst of dinner or a party—even in the very middle of a conversation—he would rise and dash out of the house, mumbling epithets to himself. For the most part, however, his wit and charm outweighed these momentary lapses and his family and friends chalked it all up to his genius. But now the erratic side of Jemmy's nature was becoming more noticeable. It seemed that his mind was always burning with one issue or another.

It is perhaps curious that the man Mercy chose for her husband was totally unlike her beloved brother. Warren was calm, quiet, and studious, though not an intellectual. He was what the Puritans called a man of "first principles." That meant that he followed tradition and saw no reason to deviate from the common wisdom of either his church or his community. Mercy, of course, was equally attached to "first principles" because of her training and unwavering faith in God and religion. However, her wide reading had given her a more philosophical inclination based on the growing eighteenth-century creed of egalitarianism, which she extended not only to politics but to her personal life as a wife and mother. She later wrote that she was "stimulated to observation by a mind that had not yielded to the assertion that all political attentions lay out of the road of female life." James noted that she had "a woman's temperament and a man's mind," which may have been a bit of a left-handed compliment, but it was accurate in emphasizing Mercy's dual nature, so unusual for a woman of her time.

It would be a few years before her political side would show itself, but as a woman her philosophy was put immediately into practice. Mercy was a superb household manager, partly out of training and inclination, and also because a house run like clockwork left its mistress free, as she said, for "the book and the pen." Obviously she gave no thought to abandoning her studies just because she had married, and apparently, James was in agreement. Warren's considerable wealth allowed Mercy to make the family library one of the largest in Massachusetts. Their first three years of marriage were passed in quiet prosperity, Mercy copying and mastering the styles of her favorite poets, James managing the Eel River farm. Their first child, whom they named James, was not born until 1757. Four more sons would follow in the next nine years. It seemed an ideal life, but events were already set in motion that would change it radically.

By 1760 many Americans became concerned with the coercive and even repressive measures that the British had enforced on the colonies in order to conduct the French and Indian War. There was increased taxation levied directly by Parliament and, perhaps most intolerable of all, the writs of assistance by which a British customs agent could inspect private property at will and press it and its owner into involuntary service. The current writs were due to expire in 1761 and needed to be reapproved by the Massachusetts Council to remain as law.

A group of sixty-three Boston merchants signed a petition requesting that the writs not be merely considered by the council, but that their legality be tested in court. Chief Justice Hutchinson consented and by all rights, Jemmy, who now held the post of king's advocate as prosecuting attorney for the province, should have pleaded the government side. The merchants, however, retained him as their counsel and Jemmy resigned his position as advocate to take the case. His old mentor, Jeremiah Gridley, was appointed in his place. The stage was set for the first real battle of the Revolution.

Gridley argued for the writs purely on the basis of statute and precedence, but when Jemmy finally arose, the court heard the first major attack on British sovereignty conducted on philosophical grounds. He spoke eloquently for four straight hours, denying the power of Parliament to impose writs or taxes without the consent of colonial legislatures. His argument began by reference to Locke's notions of natural rights and self-evident truths and concluded with an historical examination of the English Constitution. Jemmy built to a crescendo that enraptured the audience; for the first time, he spoke the words that would ring throughout the 1760s: "Taxation without representation is tyranny." In the back of the room a young barrister, John Adams, was spending his first day in court. A few years later he would comment, "Otis was a flame of fire. Then and there was the first scene of the first act of opposition to the arbitrary claims of Great Britain. Then and there the child independence was born."

Hutchinson and Gridley pointed out that Otis's case did not pertain to the fact of law, but was rather an historical and philosophical argument. With support gathering behind Jemmy, however, Hutchinson refused to make a decision and sloughed the case off onto the courts in London. The decision came back within a few months and, not surprisingly, it upheld the writs. The result was that, even in defeat, Jemmy emerged as the hero. Three months later on a wave of anti-British sentiment, he was swept into the General Court where he would serve for the next several years. There he became a most formidable symbol of opposition, and his actions in the court were directly influential in bringing on the ultimate confrontation of war.

In 1757 the Warrens had purchased and moved to a large house in the town of Plymouth. The Eel River farm was retained; they would use it as a sort of summer home. Mercy had loved the rural isolation of the farm, but it was too solitary an environment for a woman who had so much to share with the world. Now she felt the need of coming in contact with other minds. Plymouth was a small town, but it was on a crossroads leading from Boston and a constant stream of visitors passed through. For this reason the Warrens also thought that it would be a better place to raise children, for they would have access to a wider range of people and ideas.

James and Mercy were both lenient in their child rearing. The old obligations to duty and a love of books and learning certainly had to be instilled, but as Mercy saw it, these were to be accomplished by the force of pure reason. Although the Warren boys were rarely disciplined, they were constantly subjected to their mother's lengthy discourses, warning them of the pitfalls of life and advising them in a highly philosophical manner. This she continued long after they had grown and moved away from home.

Perhaps she had talked the boys out by the time they came of age, for none of them became especially distinguished, almost as if they had given up trying to match their mother's formidable talents. The second son, Winslow, was by far Mercy's favorite, and though he would show many of the sparks of genius of both Mercy and Jemmy, his life was erratic and, ultimately, wasted. There was much sadness in store for Mercy's family and now, from Plymouth, she watched the unfolding of the last act in the brilliant career of her brother.

Jemmy was often called upon to take one extreme stand or another. When he attempted to reconcile opposing views, it was inevitable that he would come under attack from both sides. The constant controversy did little for his equilibrium. And in 1764 Jemmy was back in the fray against his old enemies. Fighting the Grenville Act, which placed an external tax on molasses, and then in 1765 arguing against the Stamp Act, he was unsparing in his vilification of Bernard, the new royal governor of Massachusetts, and Hutchinson. In fact there were many, even among his followers, who felt that he might be hurting the colonial cause by the violence of his outbursts. Samuel Adams was alarmed because, for all his agitation, he hoped for a peaceful separation of England and her colonies.

The same year as the Stamp Act crisis, Jemmy had written a pamphlet entitled "Rights of the British Colonies Asserted and Proved." It was a call for political and economic self-determination and, in a rather conciliatory manner, left open the possibility of Parliament's sovereignty. Its influence was immediately felt as it was read widely both in America and England.

By 1769 the situation in the colonies had taken on major crisis proportions. New taxes, writs of assistance, and antidissent laws were imposed and led the General Court to all but open warfare against Hutchinson and Bernard. Jemmy seemed to have abandoned reason altogether and now was in a constant and alarming rage. He monopolized the conversation wherever he went, as Samuel Adams sadly noted, "in an unpleasant way, showing no politeness nor delicacy, no learning nor ingenuity, no taste or sense." Still, Mercy was as quick to defend him as always. He was, she said, "susceptible of quick feelings and warm passions," and she felt that his "ebullitions of zeal . . . betrayed him into unguarded epithets." But Mercy was being kind; actually Jemmy's passions were leading him to the brink.

The final blow, it seems, came in late 1769. In the wake of riots and general anarchy, British troops were brought into Boston. Mercy later echoed her brother's sentiments: "The experience of all ages shows that a standing army is the most ready engine in the hand of despotism." In the ensuing conflict over the removal of the troops, Bernard dissolved the General Court and promptly departed for England, leaving Hutchinson as acting governor. This was too much for Jemmy Otis. Brandishing a cane, he stormed into a known Loyalist coffeehouse and was beaten senseless with a bludgeon of some kind. He was brought home later that evening with a deep gash in his head, mumbling incoherently.

Jemmy recovered, but the wound to his head did little for his already faltering mind. Within a few months he attempted to return to Boston politics, but was subject to what his friends called his "mad frieks," both in his own home and in public. An entry in Hutchinson's diary in 1771 told the story succinctly: "Otis was carried off today in a post chaise, bound hand and foot. He has been as good as his word, set the Province in flame and perished in the attempt." Jemmy spent the next twelve years at Barnstable and Andover where he descended deeper into insanity, yet becoming remarkably calm, almost pitifully calm as one of his friends put it, "like a lamb."

Mercy rarely mentioned her brother after this, as if she could not detract in the slightest way from Jemmy's glory in the 1760s. But his actions and his ruin left behind a firm resolve in Mercy's mind. Now as the events of the early seventies sped on, she would take her revenge and continue her brother's cause in the best way she knew how. Writing of Hutchinson's arrogance up to the time of the Boston Tea Party of 1773 and of his refusal to take the pending revolution seriously, she wrote that he "gave a fair opening to the friends of their country which they did not neglect" the result being that he "fanned rather than checked the *amor patriae* characteristic of the times." When Hutchinson left for England in 1774 never to return to his homeland again, Mercy cheered silently and felt some pride in having been instrumental in blocking his control of the province. Her campaign for American independence had already begun. When the news arrived shortly thereafter that the Massachusetts charter—the last hope of the colonialists—was to be broken, it was with resolve and a backward glance to Jemmy's efforts that Mercy wrote, "The ball of empire rolled westward. The painful period hastened on, when the connexion which nature and interest had long maintained between Great Britain and the colonies must be broken off; the sword drawn, and the scabbard thrown down the gulf of time."

If James Otis was the first and greatest influence on Mercy's life and writing, John Adams was the second. He had met the Warrens sometime in 1767 while riding circuit as a lawyer in the Plymouth area, and the three quickly became close friends. Adams's wife Abigail did not meet the Warrens until three years later when she and Mercy established a lasting, close relationship.

Little is known of these early days of the Adams-Warren friend-ship except that their minds were all traveling in the same direction. The Warrens' house at Plymouth had become an assembly place for the dissident faction in Boston, and the Adamses, Hancock, and others were regular visitors. Mercy and Abigail were privy to the ongoing discussion of politics, since both of them were considered intellectuals by their husbands and their close circle of friends. It seems that at one of these evening discussions in October 1772, James Warren conceived the idea of the committees of correspondence—those groups which kept news and patriotic opin-ions circulating throughout the colonies. That same year, a lengthy poem titled "The Squabble of the Sea Nymphs" appeared in the Boston *Gazette*. Its author, Mercy Warren, had written it at the suggestion of John Adams. It blatantly satirized the British military.

Up to this time, Mercy had limited herself to writing poetry; although in the future she would occasionally return to verse, it wasn't her best work. Some lines from a poem written later to her husband called "To Fidelio" are typical.

> Long life I ask and blessings to descend
> And crown the efforts of my constant friend;
> My early wish and evening prayer the same,
> That virtue, health, and peace, and honest fame
> May hover o'er thee till time's latest hour. . . .

Now "The Squabble" put a different idea into Mercy's mind. The realization that she could write satire, and especially that this satire could be directed to some useful end, tended to change her view of what was appropriate subject matter for a woman writer. Where her poetry had been largely imitative of Pope and Dryden, now she changed to blank verse in the style of Shakespeare and Molière, adding flourishes that were all her own.

In 1772 a satiric play was published anonymously in the *Massa-chusetts Spy*. Its full title was, *The Adulateur: A Tragedy; As It Is Now Acted In Upper Servia*. Its principal characters were Rapatio, the evil ruler of Upper Servia who intended to crush the "ardent love of liberty in Servia's free-born sons," and Brutus, the true patriot and man of conscience who must overthrow Rapatio. The work was Mercy's, of course, and Rapatio and Brutus were thinly disguised versions of Hutchinson and Jemmy Otis. The piece was used by the Patriots as propaganda, and "Rapatio" and "Caesar" became common names for the royal governor.

The following year Mercy anonymously published her second satiric drama, this time in the Boston *Gazette*. *The Defeat* again featured Rapatio and Brutus and was rushed into print in pamphlet form, probably by John Adams, and distributed as far south as Philadelphia. The play has a happy ending; the Hutchinson charac-ter is defeated as indeed the real Hutchinson appeared to be at the time. Benjamin Franklin, then the American envoy to England, had managed to intercept some of Hutchinson's letters to his brother-in-law, which adequately demonstrated Hutchinson's rath-er callous disregard for colonial grievances. Contrary to Franklin's wishes, Samuel Adams had them published in the *Gazette* and whatever hopes Hutchinson had for quieting the growing rebellion disappeared. *The Defeat* was an instant success and served to finalize the Massachusetts Patriots' commitment to overthrowing Hutchinson's government. As the evil Rapatio was made to say:

> I tremble at the purpose of my soul.
> The wooden latchet of my door ne'er clicks
> But that I start—and ask—does Brutus enter?

Brutus, of course, was gone from the scene. It was Brutus's sister that Rapatio had most to fear.

When Hutchinson departed for England in 1774, he was replaced by General Gage and Boston formally became an occupied city. Gage was never as unpopular with the Patriots as was Hutchinson, but the die had already been cast and it appeared to all that war must be imminent. In April 1775 just before the Battle of Lexington, Mercy published her third and final satire which accurately prophe-sied the coming of war. *The Group* was by far her best and most popular play. It came out in pamphlet form in two installments and quickly circulated throughout the colonies.

Few people in Boston had ever seen a play because of the stringent blue laws that forbade such things. Mercy's plays, therefore, were meant to be read and were unhampered by any restraints that the necessity of performance might place on them. A stage direction from *The Group* is telling:

> The Group [Hutchinson and his henchmen again] enter attended by a swarm of court sycophants, hungry harpies, and unprincipled danglers . . . hovering over the stage in the shape of locusts, led by Massachusettensis in the form of a basilisk; the rear brought up by Proteus, bearing a torch in one hand and a powder flask in the other, the whole supported by a mighty army and navy from Blunderland, for the laudable purpose of enslaving its best friends.

The play leveled its main attack on the American-born Loyalists (as symbolized by Hutchinson), who were shown as traitors to their own country, and against any and all Americans who vacillated in their loyalties. Mercy avenged her brother's treatment in a most effective way.

The plays had been published anonymously for two reasons: one, the common-sense fear of recriminations, and secondly, because women simply did not write satires, especially such brutal attacks on established government. Apparently, the Massachusetts Patriots were not of the same opinion, however, for they soon learned the name of the author and showered her with praise. With her fame growing beyond all normal boundaries for a respectable lady, Mercy began to have second thoughts about her role as a satirist. She wrote to John Adams.

> Personal reflections and sarcastic reproaches have generally been decryed by the wise and the worthy, both in their conversation and writings. And though a man may be greatly criminal in his conduct towards the society in which he lives. How far, sir, do you think it justifiable for any individual to hold him up the object of public derision.

> But though from the particular circumstances of our unhappy time, a little personal acrimony might be justifiable in your sex, must not the female character suffer . . . if she indulges her pen to paint in the darkest shades, even those whose vice and venality have rendered contemptible.

> Your undisguised sentiments on these points will greatly oblige a
> person who is sometimes doubtful whether the solicitations of a
> friend may not lead her to indulge a satirical propensity that ought to
> be reined in with the utmost care and attention.

Adams quickly replied from his house at Braintree, reassuring her of
her right to expose the truth and expressing great praise for her
talent. His assurances not only firmed her resolve as a writer, but
assuaged whatever doubts she might have had about the propriety
of this, her greatest pleasure.

Now although war was coming and she was deeply involved in her
writing, Mercy's sense of duty toward her family never suffered
because of other concerns. As she would continue to insist in the
future, she still emulated the simple virtues of the good wife and
mother. However, as a passionate lover of liberty and virtue, it was
impossible for her to sit on the sideline while her husband and their
friends fought for the cause of freedom. Though she called her
writing "the amusement of solitude, when every active member of
the society was engaged either in the field, or the cabinet, to resist
the strong hand of foreign domination," it was clear that, in service
of the cause, it was much more than amusement.

After the battles at Lexington and Concord, the Patriots of Boston
began fleeing that town, fearful of recriminations from the British
command. Among them, of course, were John Adams and John
Hancock who were already being sought by General Gage. They
traveled to Philadelphia where the First Continental Congress was
convened on May 10, and in a move, probably headed by Adams,
George Washington was commissioned commander in chief of the
Continental army. As head of the local committee of correspondence, James Warren departed Plymouth for Concord to aid in the
plans for an assault on British-held Boston. For the next six years he
would see little of his home or his family.

When Washington arrived to establish his winter headquarters at
Watertown, seven miles from Boston, he immediately appointed
Warren the paymaster general of the army and commissioned him
with the rank of major general. This task was an unenviable one,
however, since funds were never sufficient for keeping Washington's army together. Warren was to achieve glory in another area,
however. He had urged the establishment of a navy and was duly
put in charge of securing and outfitting coastal privateers to prey on
the British navy.

With her husband gone, Mercy tried to keep up her spirits as best she could. She and her second oldest son, Winslow, decided that they would continue to run the Eel River farm in James's absence, though Mercy turned out to be rather inept as a farmer, and Winslow simply wasn't interested. Warren would return from time to time to see his well-managed fields slowly going to seed.

In the first days of war, Mercy tended to brood. "Naked and undisciplined as we are," she wrote her husband, "without experience or allies, what have we not to fear from the mighty hand of power, without principle, justice, or humanity?" She soon wrote to her husband, who was thinking of leading the next campaign into New York:

> How earnestly did I ever entreat my dear Mr. Warren not to accept of an appointment which my foreboding heart intimated would involve me in the depths of distress? With my eyes now swimming in tears do I recollect how many honourable, how many profitable, and how many useful employments you have refused, and accepted of this one which, whenever it was named, was a dagger to my bosom! I hardly know what I write.

As it turned out, Warren was much too busy with his duties as paymaster and on the navy board to engage in any military campaigns, but Mercy's fears never abated and were largely responsible for Warren's rather low profile in the war effort. In 1779 when it appeared that he would be chosen as a delegate to the Continental Congress, the state of Mercy's nerves was one of his principal reasons for declining. He wrote her that her "brilliant and busy imagination . . . commands admiration but is often mischievous, and when yours is not directed to the bright side of things, I often wish it as sluggish as my own." He concluded, "I wish to banter and laugh you out of your whimsical gloom." Alone with her children at Plymouth, Mercy's forebodings and "palpitating heart" often brought her to the edge of despair.

Letters and occasional visits between Mercy and Abigail Adams helped to preserve both their spirits during the long years of the war. Their rapport extended to all their interests, but they especially delighted in their intellectual companionship. Their letters were seldom without what Mercy called, "a little seasoning of politics," as well as domestic news of absent husbands, sick children, or the price of linen and cambric. They would exchange favorite books and then deliver lengthy critiques on them.

By now Mercy was familiar with a wide range of historical, political, and literary works printed in the English language. Her poetry and satirical writing had given her an inside view of the process of literary creation, and her correspondence with highly articulate people like John Adams had honed her skill at expressing herself to a fine edge. She harbored the opinion that the writing of history was the highest form of literary art, and so now she sought a new direction for her talents. She would be aided in this by a most able teacher.

Mercy, like most other educated people of her day, was familiar with the work of Catharine Macaulay, one of England's foremost writers and certainly the most celebrated woman writer in the world. Her major opus was the monumental *History of England from the Accession of James I to that of the Brunswick Line,* a liberal—some said radical—interpretation of the reign of the Stuarts. An outspoken Patriot, she had advocated American independence for several years. She had kept abreast of events and personalities in the colonies throughout the 1760s, and James Otis had not gone unnoticed by the historian. In 1769 she sent him the first volume of her *History,* inscribing it: "To you, sir, as one of the most distinguished of the great guardians of American Liberty, I offer a copy of this book." Mercy's first correspondence with Mrs. Macaulay came in 1771 when she informed her of her brother's mental collapse. The two stayed in close contact during the years that followed.

Catharine Macaulay's correspondence was so encouraging that shortly after *The Group* was published in late 1775, Mercy determined to write her own history. It would tell the story of the American Revolution from those first days of rebellion in the 1760s to the inevitable termination of the war. It would do so from the viewpoint of the conflicts and oppositions that were inherent in man's moral nature. Mercy saw man as basically moral and noble, which qualities led him to throw off the yoke of tyranny as the Americans were currently doing. While man's reason and conscience led him to this elevated state of affairs, however, it also led him to establish new bases of power and wealth—both of which inevitably corrupted him. Only a firm reliance on divine guidance could keep men from irreversible corruption. These themes would run throughout Mercy's work and, due to the struggles for power that followed the war, they would lead her to extend her *History* through the periods of the Confederation and the first three presidential administrations.

Writing history was a bold step, however, and Mercy was still sensitive to any suggestion that she was being improper or unfeminine. In her introduction to the work she acknowledged that "it is true that there are certain appropriate duties assigned to each sex; . . . yet recollecting that every domestic enjoyment depends on the unimpaired possession of civil and religious liberty, . . . the work was not relinquished." Once again, it was John Adams who reassured her. "If the fair should be excused from the arduous cares of war and state," he wrote to James Warren, then surely Mercy and Abigail were exceptions because "I have ever ascribed to those two ladies, a share and no small one neither, in the conduct of our American affairs."

The task of gathering materials and writing took up much of Mercy's time while her husband was away at war, and the size and difficulty of the project often depressed her. She would work at it sporadically for the next thirty years, setting it aside at least twice, once when the war was going badly for the Americans in 1778 and 1779 and again through most of the 1780s when party strife between Federalist and anti-Federalist factions threatened to tear the country apart.

Surprisingly, as Mercy began to grapple with her *History,* she still found time to serve the cause as a playwright. The British had been defeated at the Battle of Saratoga in the fall of 1777, and their officers, including General "Gentleman Johnny" Burgoyne, had been installed in Boston for the winter, technically as prisoners of war. In fact they lived riotously, giving balls and parties and presenting plays despite the blue laws. Burgoyne, himself an accomplished writer, wrote and produced a play called *The Blockade of Boston* which ridiculed the Patriots. A copy of the script promptly ended up in Mercy's hands at Plymouth and her reply was ready within a few months.

Mercy turned to farce to make her point. *The Blockheads* presented a portrait of Burgoyne and his troops, cringing in Boston, waiting for spring and transport back to England. It worked admirably as a piece of Patriot propaganda, though one surprising quality is its extremely coarse prose dialogue. Mercy apparently had no more fears about the propriety of satirical writing. At one point a timorous British soldier expresses his trepidation: "I would rather s--t my breeches than go without these forts to ease myself." The American soldiers loved the dialogue in *The Blockheads.* It seems that with all of her fine upbringing, Mercy had managed also to learn the coarser ways of the world. She was careful, though, not to have her name associated with the play. Although she made British soldiers talk like British soldiers, having it officially known that she was the author of those words was quite a different matter.

After the success of *The Blockheads,* Mercy returned to her *History,* but she was still to write one last satirical play in response to a burning issue of the war period. By 1779 the war had shifted to the South, and the merchants and upper classes of Boston were making fortunes in supplying provisions. Along with this went a gaudy life-style that appalled Patriots such as the Warrens and the Adamses.

To Mercy this behavior constituted a call to arms and her satirical pen was once again set in motion. *The Motley Assembly,* published in 1779, was perhaps the first American play to contain only American characters. It was short, written in prose dialogue, and probably her best effort up to that time. It was a brilliant attack on the Loyalists of Boston, and it reserved its harshest criticism for the American turncoats who looked for a return to British rule because of the elegant social atmosphere that would accompany it. It condemned profiteering and any show of Anglophilism among the Americans. Once again, it was an immediate success and was circulated throughout the colonies.

In 1781, that most decisive year of the war, Cornwallis had been defeated at Yorktown, and the Americans awaited the finalization of the peace—a process that would take still another two years. Congress immediately began to cut back its war-related expenditures, and one of the first things to go was Warren's navy. For James, however, this seemed auspicious. He was a passionate farmer who had been kept from his fields too long, and to make things better, Thomas Hutchinson's magnificent plantation, Milton Hill, was for sale. Ironically, almost seven years to the day that their old enemy sailed for England, the Warrens with their youngest son George moved to Milton, only fourteen miles from Boston.

James's reasons for removing to Milton were threefold. First, he would establish the great farm that had always been his dream; secondly, he would leave an impressive landed legacy to his sons; and finally, Mercy would be closer to the social and intellectual world of Boston than she had been at Eel River and Plymouth. But his dreams were never realized. Mercy remained a lonely and, at times, even introverted person; indeed it seemed to be her natural state. One by one the boys abandoned Milton, none of them showing any interest in their father's plans. James would be forced to run the farm single-handedly for almost eight years, but it would prove to be too difficult and unprofitable a task. In 1788 the Warrens would sell Milton and return to the ancestral home at Plymouth.

The Milton interlude was a time of great personal tragedy for the Warrens, especially for Mercy. James Jr. lost his leg, became extremely dejected, and wandered off to teach school in a rural district of Connecticut. Charles died in Spain after years of suffering from tuberculosis. Winslow, the favorite, for whom Mercy had had such great hopes, wandered about Europe and America running up huge personal debts. George, the youngest, became a pioneer in the wilds of Maine. Only Henry was to assume some respectability by establishing himself in a law practice at Plymouth.

In Mercy's own family the old patriarch, Colonel Otis, had died in 1781. Jemmy, now thoroughly quiescent, his mind almost completely gone, went to live with an old friend at Andover. One day he casually gathered all of his letters, documents, speeches, and books and made a huge bonfire of them. If history has often overlooked James Otis, it is probably because of this literal and symbolic immolation of the record of perhaps the most brilliant mind in the Revolution. A few weeks later Jemmy was leaning against a doorpost, looking out at a raging thunderstorm. A bolt of lightning hit the chimney, traveled down the frame of the house to the post where he was standing, and Jemmy died instantly. The last act had been written in the great Patriot's life. Surprisingly, it inspired Mercy to even greater literary triumphs in the otherwise disheartening years of the Warrens' Milton experiment.

Retreating from grief, Mercy plunged into the reading of Spanish history, probably because it was fairly exotic and had elements of the grand and tragic that she felt in her own life. Predictably, it led to more play-writing as now she had set aside her *History* once again. *The Ladies of Castile* was Mercy's first drama written in the classical style. It was as radical a change for her as the departure from poetry to satirical drama had been a decade before. Its theme, however, was still that of revolution, this time set in the days of struggle before the rise of the despotic family of Ferdinand. Its leading character, a woman named Maria, is the first great heroine in any of Mercy's work. Not surprisingly, Maria is Mercy, the wife of a Patriot and the sister of another who fights tyranny only to be overwhelmed by tragedy.

The Ladies of Castile took her about a year to write, but as soon as she had finished sometime in 1785, she immediately began to work on a second drama, *The Sack of Rome.* Historically, it was fairly straightforward; as she said in her preface, "There is but little mixture of fable in the narration." The characters, however, were brought to life for an obvious purpose. The evil Emperor, Valentinian, is pitted against rebellious citizens, led by Petronius Maximus. Valentinian's wife emerges as both a heroine and a villain. Images of George III, James Otis, and betrayers of the American Revolution abound with deeds that range from heroism to treachery. A work of great force and powerful language, it seemed to reflect Mercy's own misgivings and sense of tragedy.

All of Mercy's plays were meant to be read. As a strongly religious person, she obeyed the blue laws and publicly protested any desire to have her works performed. Her two historical dramas, however, were clearly written from the practical viewpoint of stage direction. To *The Sack of Rome* she appended the following epilogue:

> The Author asks but this small boon of you,
> Pray let it pass at least a night or two;
> And if the moral in this pious age
> Should let it live a week upon the stage;
> Some gambling fools by Maximus's fate
> Might learn their follies ere it was too late.
> Might stay at home and save their pretty spouses,
> And horns prevent by lodging at their houses.

The cat, so to speak, was out of the bag. Mercy sent a copy of the play to John Adams, now the American ambassador in London, and asked if there were any chances that he could get it produced on the London stage. Adams replied that the British were anxious to forget any and all things American, and there would be little chance of even having it published in England. And he encouraged her to return to her historical writing.

Following her old friend's advice, Mercy did return to her *History.* She must also have sensed that such extreme patriotic writing was already becoming out-of-date in 1787.

As James Warren began to see the futility of his dreams for Milton Hill, he once again plunged into politics. He ran for governor of Massachusetts in 1785 and for lieutenant governor the following year but was defeated both times. In 1787, a year before the Warrens' return to Plymouth, he ran for delegate to the Massachusetts Assembly and was elected. In the economic chaos that followed the war, the small farmers had been the hardest hit by the lack of currency, rising taxes, and, to the horror of the old Patriots, the reinstitution of debtors' prisons. As a farmer himself, Warren sympathized with them, and now being in a position of public leadership, he was outspoken in his opinions against the economic policies of the new government. Mercy and James began writing to Adams in London complaining about the situation and vilifying the courts that enforced repressive measures against poor farmers.

It was Adams's opinion that existing law, whatever its merits, must be adhered to until it could be legally changed—a strangely unrevolutionary position that showed how much his ideas had altered since the 1760s. To Adams, it seemed that the Warrens had changed, too. He refused to comment on the political content of the Warrens' letters and took a dim view of their activities. A deep rift was growing between the Warrens and the Adamses.

Actually, the break between Mercy and John Adams had been slowly growing throughout the 1780s. The correspondence between them had been lively at first, but as the decade dragged on with Adams's years of diplomatic service in Europe, he seemed to become more and more sensitive to the imagined slights of his old friends. His letters to Mercy display a bit of hurt pride when he felt that she was not writing to him often enough. In a letter to James Warren in 1782, he casually mentioned that he hoped Mercy would give a place in her *History* to his Dutch negotiations. Mercy replied bluntly that "a blank shall be left in certain annals for your Dutch negotiation, unless you condescend to furnish with your own hand a few more authentic documents." Writing to Warren in the late 1780s, Adams sounded the note of fear of a man who loathed criticism and wanted desperately to assure his place in history. "I dread her history . . ." he wrote.

The final break between the two families began in 1787 when the new Constitution was being framed. The Federalists, led by Washington, Adams, and Hamilton, were proposing a strong central government, an idea which in itself discomfitted the likes of Jefferson and the Warrens. To a large extent the provision for a division of powers dissipated this objection, but still, the proposed Constitution contained no bill of rights. The Federalists maintained that chaos would ensue if the Constitution were not immediately accepted as written, and the Adamses, recently returned from England, supported this view.

Mercy, however, could only see that the new government would not provide enough protection for the rights of the individual, and so she jumped into the fray, hurriedly producing a pamphlet entitled, *Observations on the New Constitution and on the Federal and State Conventions. By a Columbian Patriot. Sic Transit Gloria Americana.* It was Mercy at her most intellectual and didactic, and it was extremely dull. Nevertheless, it circulated throughout the new states, though it was read only by the very well educated—its elevated style was hardly of interest to the common man. Of course it came to the attention of John Adams, and to him it looked like an attack on the government he was trying to preserve.

The Constitution was finally ratified and, much to the relief of the anti-Federalists, Jefferson supplied the first ten amendments, the Bill of Rights, which were adopted by the First Congress. The union had, in fact, been preserved through the efforts and compromise of both parties, though the new vice-president, John Adams, was less than gracious toward his political opponents.

For Mercy, John Adams was still her friend, even if the relationship had become somewhat strained. She also felt that she had quite a stake in the new government, and that she and her husband had been instrumental over the years in making it possible. It was only natural that she should feel obliged to offer criticism and advice where she thought it was needed.

But Adams was becoming more sensitive where Mercy was concerned and her criticisms stung. Even Abigail, Mercy's oldest and dearest friend, wrote to her sister accusing Mercy of unbridled ambition and hoping that the Warrens and all they stood for in the anti-Federalist cause would fail. She concluded with the line, "They were my old and dear friends for whom I once entertained the highest respect." This seemingly irreconcilable rift lasted for only a brief time, since by 1790 the Warrens and Adamses were corresponding once again. It was a sad commentary on the politics of the times that differing ideologies had separated the two great families. Though their correspondence was resumed, it always lacked the vivacity and deep friendship of earlier days. For her part, Mercy had even greater reasons for maintaining a certain distance from her Federalist friends.

Under the laws of the new government no distinction was made between indebtedness and felony. The debtors' prisons had remained a common feature of American life. Mercy's beloved Winslow, now back in Boston, had run up huge debts and was accordingly thrown into jail for a month. Finally out on bond, for the first time in his life he pursued a cause and defended himself brilliantly in court, challenging the whole structure of the law that made indebtedness a crime. While awaiting an appeal, he apparently felt some remorse for a misspent life and enlisted in the army to fight against Indian uprisings on the Pennsylvania frontier. A few months later Mercy received word that her son had been killed when Indians overran the American camp. Surely, to Mercy, it must have seemed that the event which set this whole affair in motion was the application of a law with which she disagreed and which Adams backed. The experience was such a wrenching one for Mercy that she discontinued work on her history, and little was heard from her throughout the rest of the 1790s.

Nor could she rouse herself in 1796 when John Adams was elected president and established that most Federalist of all regimes. There was a note from Mercy late in his administration praising him for his negotiations with the new French government, but otherwise there was silence. The death of her son and, seemingly, the death of her ideal of government coincided, and a pall settled on her life.

However, 1800 brought a great surprise to both the Warrens and the Adamses. Adams was defeated by Jefferson, who swept into office with all of the anti-Federalist ideas that he and the Warrens had cherished for so many years. The Warrens had backed Jefferson ever since the mid-eighties and now James sent his congratulations to the new president. Jefferson responded, thanking them for their faith and support, noting especially of Mercy: "I pray you to present my homage of my great respect to Mrs. Warren. I have long possessed evidence of her high station in the ranks of genius and have considered her silence a proof that she did not go with the current." It was a jubilant time for the Warrens that began to pull Mercy out of her doldrums, even though their "proper place in society" would never be fully restored in Boston, which remained Federalist.

Tragedy was still a significant part of Mercy's life in 1800. Word arrived from Maine that her youngest son, George, had died of pneumonia on the northern frontier. But the remaining son, Henry, was now a clerk in the state legislature, and he visited Plymouth often, providing encouragement.

For the next five years, Mercy worked continuously on the *History*. The final volume was finished and the set was published in 1805 when Mercy was seventy-seven years old. No one was spared in

the intense biographical portraits that were the most outstanding
feature of the work. Such was her consistency and dedication to
those "first principles" that not only did the British feel the barb of
her pen, but also those Americans who, she felt, betrayed the
Revolution or used it for their own personal gains.

The Federalists, among all Americans, were treated to Mercy's
harshest critique. Nor did she spare her old friend, John Adams.
Mercy offered some praise where it was due, though her consistent
anti-Federalist approach resulted in a searing portrait of Adams and
his administration. As letters of praise poured into Plymouth, none
appeared from Adams. The man who had heaped such extravagant
praise on Mercy over the years, and who had encouraged her to
write the *History* in the first place, made only one final comment,
and that not until 1813. In a letter to Elbridge Gerry he wrote:

> History is not the province of ladies. These three volumes neverthe-
> less contain many facts worthy of preservation. Little passions and
> prejudices, want of information, false information, want of experi-
> ence, erroneous judgment, and frequent partiality, are among the
> faults.

Now in his eighties, James Warren Sr. had continued to supervise
the Eel River farm, though severe gout often kept him confined to
the house in Plymouth. His generally good health failed in 1808,
and on November 27, Warren died at Plymouth. Soon after a letter
arrived from Samuel Mitchill in Washington, dated the day before
Warren's death:

> Madam,—As one of the joint committee appointed by the two houses
> of congress to provide books for their library, I do myself the pleasure
> of acknowledging the receipt of your history of the rise, progress and
> termination of the American revolution. By some oversight of the
> committee, it had happened, that your excellent performance had
> not been purchased. It has therefore arrived in good season and is the
> more acceptable to us. And they who search this collection, for the
> history of their country, will be sure to find the volumes of Mrs.
> Warren on the same shelf, with those of Gordon, Ramsay, and
> Marshall.

It was almost a maxim of Mercy's life that triumph and tragedy
came together, though now, in old age, it did not inspire her to new
literary production. Sad resignation over the loss of her husband

was mingled with a feeling of accomplishment and a life well spent in service to the religious and philosophical ideals that she had formulated so many years before. Her remaining years were to be spent happily and peacefully at Plymouth.

The War of 1812 prompted a burst of correspondence from Mercy, but she and the Adamses only evaluated the state of affairs. Before Mercy would have been furiously involved in writing patriotic propaganda. To her it was only one more sad proof of what her *History* stressed over and over again—that the defense of the liberties that the Revolution had been fought for would have to be an ongoing process for future generations of Americans. The old Puritan notions of the basic imperfections of man were borne out once again.

Mercy's final letters to John Adams came in August 1814. They showed that she had kept up with things quite well for a woman of eighty-six. The first was on August 4:

Do you remember who was the author of a little pamphlet entitled *The Group?* . . . A friend of mine who lately visited the Athenaeum saw it among a bundle of pamphlets, with a high encomium of the author, who, as he asserted, was Mr. Samuel Barrett. You can, if you please, give a written testimony contradictory of the false assertion.

On the eleventh she wrote again:

If the author of *The Group* ever deserved half the encomiums you have lavished on her talent, it ought to be rescued from oblivion. This little work was committed to the press by yourself the winter before Lexington Battle.

Adams's reply was his final one to Mercy:

What brain could ever have conceived or suspected Samuel Barrett, Esq., to have been the author of *The Group?* . . . There was but one person in the world, male or female, who could, at that time, in my opinion, have written it; and that person was Madam Mercy Warren, the historical, philosophical, poetical, and satirical consort of the Colonel, since General James Warren of Plymouth, sister of the great but forgotten James Otis.

A more accurate summary of Mercy's life could not have been written. Her brother Jemmy, her enlightened husband, and her own belief that the career of wife and mother need not relegate women to a subordinate position—all of these had combined to produce an intriguing and fruitful life. As one writer has said of her, Mercy Otis Warren did not agitate for women's rights, she simply lived as if she had them. On October 19, 1814 she died quietly at her home in Plymouth.

7

Jane Franklin Mecom

ON MARCH 12, 1712 the last of Josiah Franklin's seventeen children came squalling into the world at the small, wood frame house at the corner of Union and Hanover Streets in Boston. It was a girl, the last of seven, whom Josiah and his wife named Jane after one or another of the several Janes in their families. The mother, Abiah Folger Franklin, looked up from her bed in gratitude at the strong limbs and healthy color of her new daughter, for she herself was sick and exhausted. She was Josiah's second wife and had borne ten of the children in rapid succession. This coupled with years of near-poverty conditions had not helped her constitution, so her health began to decline.

Overhanging the Franklins' house was the sign of the Blue Ball, and downstairs Josiah labored at his trade. He was a tallow chandler; that is, he made soap and candles. Among the articles he made and sold was the famous Crown Soap, the manufacture of which was a carefully guarded secret. The business was a flourishing one by small tradesmen's standards, and Josiah had even held a number of minor public posts in Boston over the years, but his income was always strained by the size of his family. If it was not exactly poverty that the Franklins lived in, neither was there always adequate provision for food, clothing, and winter heat. The cramped quarters of the small house also led to the easy communication of disease and the desire on the part of the children to leave home at an early age.

Three sons had died in infancy; a fourth had drowned in a tub of soap water before he was two. Three brothers and four sisters married before Jane was four, and one brother had been lost at sea. Another went to London to become a printer's apprentice. By the time Jane was old enough to remember, there were never more than three other children in the house at any one time—her next oldest sister, Lydia, a dull and unimaginative girl; a much older sister, Sarah, who was burdened with the housework and the care of their sickly mother; and most important of all, her brother Benjamin, six years her senior.

Jane's life would be similar to that of her parents. She had too many children and experienced much personal tragedy—even abject poverty. As the Revolution approached and progressed, she would not become a great heroine or statesman's wife. She would, however, leave a sophisticated appreciation of the momentous questions of the era in her letters to her brother. The rich intimacy and mutual respect that developed early between Jane and Benjamin led to this close relationship and the truly amazing correspondence between them. Jane, therefore, must be seen as an important figure in America's struggle for independence, for through her life and letters we gain new perspectives on both the Revolution and the career of her brilliant brother.

There is no direct evidence that Jane ever went to school, though a letter written to her by Ben many years later referred to "an ancient poet whose works we have all studied and copied at school long ago." Her competence in a variety of areas also indicates that perhaps she did attend one of the small private schools for tradesmen's children. There she probably learned the basic rudiments of reading, writing, and the compilation of household accounts, in addition to needlework and embroidery.

In the Franklin home she learned the domestic crafts, including the dying and weaving of wool and cotton and the secret of the Franklin soap. From her later writing it is evident that she learned to read all the books and papers available in the house, including the ledgers of the family business, many pamphlets and sermons, as well as the copybooks accumulated in the education of her many brothers. Benjamin went to George Brownell's school on Hanover Street from the time Jane was four, and taught his alert little sister some of the things he learned there. As was typical for girls of her position at that time, she learned little of the outside world and was entirely untrained in languages. She was apologetic all her life for her inadequate training in spelling and composition.

Nevertheless, Jane was a fast learner and was apparently possessed of singularly clear judgment even as a young girl. Compared to the other girls in the family, she was also rather vivacious and pretty. It seems that Jane and Benjamin recognized a certain genius in each other and so were closer than any other members of the family. In 1727, nine years after Ben had run away from home and had served apprenticeships as a printer in London and Philadelphia, he wrote from the latter city his first letter to Jane. Referring to some information passed on by a friend, he stated, "I am highly pleased with the account Captain Freeman gives me of you. I always judged by your behavior when a child that you would make a good, agreeable woman, and you know you were ever my particular favorite." He concluded with the following passage:

> Sister, farewell, and remember that modesty, as it makes the most homely virgin amiable and charming, so the want of it infallibly renders the most perfect beauty disagreeable and odious. But when that brightest of female virtues shines among the other perfections of body and mind in the same person, it makes the woman more lovely than an angel. Excuse this freedom, and use the same with me.

Jane would cherish this letter over the years, for it signaled the beginning of her brother's sharing with her his most intimate opinions. Although heavily weighted toward traditional prudence, they bespoke a sense of conduct that was no less import to Jane.

On July 27 of that same year, Jane married Edward Mecom, a poor saddler, whose family was even more obscure than the little-known Franklins. She was barely fifteen. Two years after their marriage, Edward was chosen a clerk of the market and was becoming a modest success in the society of small tradesmen to which the Franklins had belonged. In fact, Jane and Edward had come to live with them under the sign of the Blue Ball, and here their first child, Josiah, was born. He lived barely a year. Between 1731 and 1733 two more sons, Edward and Benjamin, were born. Ben, now married three years to Deborah Read, also had two boys, William (who was illegitimate; perhaps Jane knew this, though she never mentioned it) and Francis, who would die at the age of four. Jane and Ben congratulated each other on their families and offered consolation as deaths occurred, though no correspondence between them remains from the next ten years. In that time, Jane bore five more children and, in all, she would eventually have twelve.

The early promise of success in Edward's business was slow in developing, and his meager income proved to be inadequate for his growing family. The worst blow to Jane's happiness came with the discovery of fundamental weaknesses in the bodies and minds of her children. Three of them died in infancy, and though Jane grieved, she could not consider herself exceptionally afflicted, since infant mortality was common at the time. The real tragedy lay in the poor health of those children who survived infancy. The son who had been named after his mother's illustrious brother was unstable and irresponsible and finally required confinement in an asylum. Another son, Peter, was an imbecile, incapable of caring for himself. Some of Jane's children did reach an age where marriages and careers were begun, but even these were unfortunate. Each of them in turn succumbed to illness, as did their children. Three of Jane's children, Edward, Ebeneezer, and Sarah, returned to her poor home to die, leaving spouses and sickly grandchildren.

Edward Mecom offered little in the way of support to his wife as she faced these sorrows and challenges. He was in ill health most of the time and, with the death of each child, he only fell deeper into depression. With Edward an invalid, the family income was reduced to such an extent that Jane was forced to take in boarders, adding further to her burden.

The consistent pattern of frailty apparent in the Mecom offspring indicated that there was some congenital and perhaps even hereditary problem. People living during the eighteenth century tended to take a rather unscientific view of such a situation, and Jane's reactions to the two greatest tragedies of her life amply demonstrate this viewpoint.

After lingering for several years in generally poor health, Edward died in September 1765. Jane's entry in her "Book of Ages"—the little copybook where she recorded births and deaths in the family—reads as follows: "God sees meet to follow me with Repeeted corections this morning 3 oclock Died my husband in a Stedy hope of a happy hear after." Writing two weeks later to Ben's wife, Deborah, Jane noted: "Nothing but trouble can you hear from me, but I do my endeavor to adopt the great Pope's doctrine with regard to the Providence of God: 'Whatever is, is right.' In a few days after I wrote my last to you it pleased God to call my husband out of this troublesome world where he had enjoyed little and suffered much by sin and sorrow."

Jane never explained this comment, though it seems to indicate that she traced her family's weakness to some sinfulness in their paternal ancestry. The Puritan mind could be harsh about such things, and she probably shared with many of her contemporaries and certainly with her brother, the belief that ambition, hard work and faith in divine providence would surely result in prosperity. Since her marriage had not prospered, though she herself had all the essential qualities and virtues, she probably felt that the sin was her husband's. Though her own brothers and sisters fared little better than her children, Jane apparently never imagined that the "sin" might exist on both sides of the family. She never blamed herself for her children's tragically short and twisted lives.

The second blow came two years later. Jane had hoped that her youngest child, Polly, would be spared the misery which had afflicted the rest of the family. Polly was the brightest of the children and had a gentle, teasing wit which lightened the dreary atmosphere of the Mecom household. By the time she reached adolescence, there were always grieving wives and sickly grandchildren present for whom the young girl cared. Jane found that, of all the children, Polly alone shared with her the same spirited approach to life. Apparently Polly responded in kind to her mother's affection, helping and pleasing as none of the others could through the family's most difficult times.

In 1767, however, when Polly was nineteen, Jane found that she too was growing weak and decided that, at any cost, this child must be saved. Polly was sent to live with cousins at Nantucket in the hope that the healthy climate, away from the darkened Mecom household, would help her regain her strength. But Polly declined rapidly at Nantucket and was dead and buried before her mother even heard the news. After years of bearing children, caring for them through their often short lives of illness, and watching as each of them died in turn, the pain at this loss of her favorite daughter was almost more than she could bear. She cried out in anguish to the only person who fully understood the misery of her last forty years as a wife and mother. Her first letter after Polly's death was to Benjamin.

> Sorrows roll upon me like waters of the sea. I am hardly allowed time to fetch my breath. I am broken with breach upon breach, and I have now, in the first flow of my grief, been almost ready to say, "What have I more?" But God forbid that I should indulge in that thought though I have lost another child. God is sovereign, and I submit.

This lamentation could not have done other than move her brother. Yet Benjamin realized that far less tragedy had resulted in the collapse of even stronger individuals, and so his reply was a careful expression of sympathy and understanding calculated to quiet her more passionate emotions. He mentioned that he had suffered a similar loss in the death of his son, Francis, and had found time alone the only means of dulling the edge of grief.

> The longer we live, we are exposed to more of these strokes of Providence; but though we consider them as such, and yet know it is our duty to submit to the Divine Will, yet when it comes our turn to bear what so many millions after us must bear, we are apt to think our case particularly hard, consolations however kindly administered seldom afford us any relief, natural affections will have their course, and time proves our best comforter.

Part of the reason for the highly rational tone of this response was the fact that Benjamin was clearly of a more secular mind than was Jane. While she took the view of pious resignation, he felt that the passage of life was simply a natural fact, perhaps even divorced from any direct intervention on the part of a supreme God. He would not have said this to Jane, however, for he knew her to be a deeply religious person. Rather, he relied upon her remarkable sense of proportion and emotional stability. He knew that every argument which might lessen her grief had already suggested itself, and so he offered only the most simple and straightforward consolations. As he was now the American envoy to Great Britain, he quickly changed the subject in response to one of her earlier requests for some of his political writings.

> You desire me to send you all the political pieces I have been author of. I have never kept them. They were most of them written occasionally for transient purposes, and having done their business they die and are forgotten. I could as easily make a collection for you of all the past parings of my nails. But I will send you what I write hereafter, and I now enclose you the last piece of mine that is printed.

The pamphlet he sent, entitled *On Smuggling,* urged the Americans to the lawful conduct of business despite repressive tax measures enacted by the British Parliament. Its clear logic and reasoned position impressed Jane; perhaps it even drew her attention from her grief, for over the past few years she had tried to sublimate her family problems with a growing interest in her brother's activities. It was not merely pride in Benjamin or curiosity over his affairs, but a genuine interest in the political turmoil that was developing around both of them. Jane's concern with her personal sorrows was soon to be replaced by events and issues of much greater magnitude.

Jane had watched with pride as Benjamin rose mightily in Philadelphia society and politics. His almanac and his profitable publishing and printing businesses were well known throughout the colonies. He had been instrumental in establishing a library and a fire department, had invented the "Pennsylvania Fireplace," was postmaster of Philadelphia, clerk of the Pennsylvania Assembly, and was in the process of forming an American Philosophical Society. During a brief visit to his sister in Boston in 1743, he observed the electrical experiments of Adam Spencer; these would soon lead Franklin to one of his most impressive accomplishments. In 1757 he would go to London as agent for the Pennsylvania Assembly for a period of five years, and in 1765 he would go to England once again until the approaching war would force his return.

Josiah and Abiah Franklin died in 1744 and 1752, respectively. The Blue Ball was sold, and Jane and her family bought a smaller boardinghouse on Hanover Street, probably with Benjamin's help. A letter from him shortly thereafter expressed this wish to his sister: "As our number grows less, let us love one another proportionately more." It was a wish that Jane echoed, and it foretold their intimacy in the years to come.

Jane's earliest surviving letter to her brother was written on December 30, 1765, shortly after the death of her husband. Edward Mecom had died intestate and so, as a matter of course, his estate went into probate. The judge of the court was Lieutenant Governor Thomas Hutchinson, who treated the widow with the utmost fairness. This same year the Stamp Act had been passed, and many of the more radical Patriots, such as James Otis and John Adams, threw the blame for this repressive measure directly on Hutchinson's shoulders. A mob had even destroyed his house, near where the Mecoms lived. Jane's letter to Ben in London was indicative of their political ideas at the time.

> The confusion and distress those oppressive acts have thrown us poor Americans into is undescribable by me, but you see the newspapers full of them. But they have fallen very short, I am told, of a description of the Lieutenant Governor's sufferings, which all circumstances considered was never equalled in any nation. . . . He is

now going from us, the greatest ornament of our country, and the most indefatigable patriot. He does me the honor to be the bearer of this, and has shown me the greatest clemency in the capacity of a judge. May God protect and preserve him still for the good of mankind, and confer on him the honor he deserves. My writing so much of the Governor at this time looks as though influenced by his goodness to me in particular, but I assure you my opinion of the gentleman was the same before I had any business with him. . . .

Hutchinson did not leave the colonies for England until 1774, and there remained several years of political and personal torment for him. In fact, he had not favored the Stamp Act. But the rabid Patriots of Boston were in no mood to quibble; where they assigned guilt, it stayed, and the Franklins' reasoned thinking on the matter was less than popular with the mob. Franklin himself was accused of favoring the Stamp Act and his family in Philadelphia was threatened. Jane wrote to Deborah:

I am amazed beyond measure . . . that your house was threatened in the tumult. I thought there had been none among you would proceed to such a length to persecute a man merely for being of the best of characters and really deserving good from the hand and tongue of all his fellow creatures. I knew there was a party that did not approve his prosecuting the business he is gone to England upon, and that some had used him with scurrilous language in some printed papers; but I was in hopes it had so far subsided as not to give you any disturbance. When I think what you must have suffered at the time, how I pity you; but I think your indignation must have exceeded your fear. What a wretched world this would be if the vile of mankind had no laws to restrain them!

The Loyalists in America were doing their best to discredit Franklin and his attempts to settle economic matters between England and the colonies, and this made his situation precarious. Nevertheless, Ben responded to Jane's indignation in his usual rational way:

I have often met with such treatment from people that I was all the while endeavoring to serve. At other times I have been extolled extravagantly where I have had little or no merit. These are the operations of nature. It sometimes is cloudy, it rains, it hails; again 'tis clear and pleasant, and the sun shines on us. Take one thing with another and the world is a pretty good sort of world, and 'tis our duty to make the best of it and be thankful.

Referring to Hutchinson, he added, "Surely the New England people, when they are rightly informed, will do justice to these gentlemen and think of them as they deserve." Ben was wrong about this, however, for Hutchinson would continue to be regarded as one of the primary villains in service to the Crown long after the Revolution was over. Franklin, however, quickly vindicated himself in his address to the House of Commons, which aided in the repeal of the Stamp Act the following year. Jane wrote offering her congratulations: "Your answers to the Parliament are thought by the best judges to exceed all that has been wrote on the subject; and being given in the manner they were are a proof that they proceeded from principle and sufficient to stop the mouths of all gainsayers." Unfortunately, Ben's rational approach to the world would not always carry the day, just as the ravings of the Massachusetts Patriots would have little influence on Jane's view of the developing crisis.

Shortly after her husband died, Jane opened a small millinery shop in Edward's old chandlery to alleviate the family's dire poverty. The goods she offered for sale—fabric, ribbons, laces, caps, and other decorative items—had been selected by Margaret Stevenson, the English society woman in whose home Benjamin lived in London. The goods were shipped across the Atlantic, either prepaid by Franklin or on consignment to Jane. In 1767, however, Boston merchants signed a nonimportation agreement to avoid British taxes, and Jane was caught in the middle with her small but thriving business. Jane wrote her brother:

> It proves a little unlucky for me that our people have taken it into their heads to be so excessive frugal at this time, as you will see by our newspapers. Our blusterers must be employed, and if they do no worse than to persuade us to "wear our old clothes over again" I can't disapprove of that in my heart; though I should like to have those that do buy and could afford it should buy what little I have to sell and employ us to make it up.

In the first blush of financial success, Jane was reluctant to see anyone's politics take it away from her. Her brother, however, had been among the pamphleteers urging the boycott, and so Jane duly paid attention to his arguments. They pointed out what she already was coming to know from her own experience: the lack of hard currency in the colonies, limitations on free importation, and high customs duties were creating a balance of trade unfavorable to

America which especially hurt the small importers like Jane. It must have been a hard decision to make—for surely there were enough Loyalists in Boston to purchase her British frivolities—but Jane renounced her foreign goods in America's interests. In January 1769 Ben wrote to her: "I should be sorry you are engaged in a business which happens not to coincide with the general interest, if you did not acquaint me that you are now near the end of it."

But this was not quite the end of it, for Jane proved to be a shrewd businesswoman. She soon discovered that she could buy her goods more cheaply at discount from Boston merchants who had already either paid the duties or had successfully smuggled in the items she wanted. Not only were her profits higher this way, but her inventory was freed from the nonimportation and purchase agreements. It is true that she assumed a rather low profile in the midst of the taxation furors in the late sixties and early seventies, but by 1773 she was running a comfortable neighborhood business on Hanover Street once again and was even back to importing goods directly from England. Benjamin, it might be added, continued to help in this regard with his London connections.

Taxation and other economic measures that had been instrumental in inflaming most of the New England Patriots seemed to have little effect on Jane's politics in the long run, though she felt the tax policies to be unfair also. With conservative Franklin practicality, she found legal ways around the measures that she knew her brother would approve of. But Jane was radicalized—in the Loyalist sense of the word—by the continual stream of abuse suffered by Benjamin at the hands of the ever-shifting American political factions. Franklin had been appointed postmaster general for all the colonies in 1754, and his enemies were fond of using this as a reason for slandering his reputation. In 1769 it was rumored that this was only the first step in his reach for power. Jane wrote that she heard he was to be appointed British under-secretary of state. Ben replied that he was too old to be "ambitious of such a station";

> But even if it were offered, I certainly would not accept it, to act under such instructions as I know must be given with it.

Ben, of course, was referring to instructions contrary to American interests.

The next year Jane heard that he had been dismissed from his office for sending letters and pamphlets to America which plainly agitated against British policies. She concluded a letter to him with the sour note, "I fancy by this time you have found there are more wicked folks in the world than you thought there was; and that they are capable of doing hurt." Once again Ben assured her that these were mere rumors, though he did note that there was some pressure for him to resign. But he wrote, "In this they are not likely to succeed, I being deficient in that Christian virtue of resignation. If they would have my office, they must take it."

Finally in 1774 Franklin was stripped of his postmaster's position. Immediately, the rumors flew that he had been fired because of incompetence. The first letter that Ben wrote after this was to his sister:

> Intending to disgrace me, they have rather done me an honor. No failure of duty in my office is alleged against me. Such a fault I should have been ashamed of. But I am too much attached to the interests of America, and an opposer of the measures of administration. The displacing me therefore is a testimony of my being uncorrupted.

It did not take long for another rumor to circulate to the effect that Franklin had actually resigned in order to take a high position in the colonial ministry from where he would enforce oppressive measures against his fellow Americans. Upon noting the charges in the American newspapers forwarded to him, Franklin hastened to write a denial to his sister:

> . . . as I am anxious to preserve your good opinion, and as I know your sentiments and that you must be much afflicted yourself, and even despise me, if you thought me capable of accepting any office from this government while it is acting with so much hostility toward my native country, I cannot miss this first opportunity to assure you that there is not the least foundation for such a report. . . . Be assured, my dear sister, that I shall do nothing to lessen myself in your esteem or my own. . . .

Jane replied with an outpouring that showed her to be solidly allied with her brother and all that he stood for:

> I think it is not profanity to compare you to Our Blessed Saviour, Who employed much of His time while here on earth in doing good to the body as well as souls of men; and I am sure I think the comparison just, often, when I hear the calumny invented and

thrown out against you while you are improving all your powers for the salvation of them very persons.

By implication, Jane could be nothing but a Patriot now, though it was clear that her loyalty to the American cause was inseparable from her loyalty to her brother.

Jane's personal circumstances had finally begun to brighten by 1769. Not only had she managed to save a little money, but her children and their families (except for one daughter) who had been taxing her resources had moved out of the small boardinghouse. At fifty-seven years of age, Jane must have experienced the first real sense of freedom in her life, and she decided to travel south to Philadelphia to see Ben's family. All along the journey she was greeted by her brother's friends and treated like an important personage. She stayed with Deborah for a few months in Philadelphia where she became affectionately known as "Aunt Mecom." On the way back to Boston she was received with great ceremony at the official residence of the governor of New Jersey—William Franklin, Ben's son. For a woman who had known only a life of poverty and pain, the new sights, the adulation and affection that were showered on her, and finally, the privileged reception at the great governor's mansion, must have been an exhilarating experience.

Upon returning to Boston, Jane found herself in the most comfortable circumstances of her life. She had a new house on Hanover Street, close to the old Blue Ball, and she was managing well with a little help from the Franklins and the small income from her business. Apparently her eyes were failing and she wrote to Ben for a pair of spectacles, perhaps even asking for the bifocals which he himself had invented. His reply is a classic which, even today, provides all the basic information for the fitting of eyeglasses.

I thought you had mentioned in one of your letters a desire to have spectacles of some sort sent to you; but I cannot find such a letter. However I send you a pair of every size glasses from 1 to 13. To suit yourself, take out a pair at a time, and hold one of the glasses first against one eye, and then against the other, looking on some small print. If the first pair suits neither eye, put them up again before you open a second. Thus you will keep them from mixing. By trying and comparing at your leisure, you may find out those that are best for you, which you cannot well do in a shop, where for want of time and care people often take such as strain their eyes and hurt them. I advise your trying each of your eyes separately, because few people's eyes are fellows, and almost everybody in reading or working uses one eye principally, the other being dimmer or perhaps fitter for distant objects, and thence it happens that the spectacles whose glasses are fellows suit sometimes that eye which before was not used, though they do not suit the other. When you have suited yourself, keep the higher numbers for future use as your eyes may grow older; and oblige your friends with the others.

People now stopped Jane at every street corner—recognizing by her spectacles that she was Ben Franklin's sister—to find out how things were going in London.

In late 1774 Jane received a letter from Ben, teasing her for her constant apologies for her writing style:

Is there not a little affectation in your apology for the incorrectness of your writing? Perhaps it is rather fishing for commendation. You write better, in my opinion, than most American women. Here indeed the ladies write generally with more elegance than the gentlemen.

Jane was no doubt pleased by this compliment from the man whose opinions she regarded most highly, but a return letter from her in November of that year contained no compliments. She sadly reported the scurrilous attacks being leveled at her former host, William Franklin.

I think it is presuming on your patience, but I must just mention the horrid lie told and published here about your son. At first it struck with a fear that it might be true, and I can't express the pain it gave me on your account; but a little consideration convinced me it was impossible, and I soon had the pleasure of hearing it contradicted.

The "horrid lie"—that William was siding with the Crown against the colonies—was unfortunately true. Father and son would irrevocably part ways within the year, and this would sadden Jane, for William was her favorite. Benjamin, no doubt, was already aware of the pending split, but as war now seemed inevitable between Britain and America, he must have regarded it stoically as one more casualty of the times. No mention was made of it in his return letter to Jane, the last he would write to her from England. Dated February 26, 1775 it bespoke Ben's habitual optimism: "I hope you continue well, as I do, thanks be to God. Be of good courage. Bad weather does not last always in any country." Two months later, while the battles at Lexington and Concord were being fought, Ben was aboard ship returning to America.

A letter written by Jane in May describing the events at Concord, probably reached Ben in Philadelphia. He could not imagine, she wrote, that

> the storm would have arisen so high as for the General [Thomas Gage] to have sent out a party to creep out in the night and slaughter our dear brethren for endeavoring to defend our own property. But God appeared for us and drove them back with much greater loss than they are willing to own. Their countenances as well as confessions of many of them shew they were mistaken in the people they had to deal with; but the distress it has occasioned is past my description. The horror the town was in when the battle approached within hearing, expecting they would proceed quite into town; the commotion the town was in after the battle ceased, by the parties coming in bringing their wounded men, caused such an agitation I believe none had much sleep. . . .

Boston had suddenly become a battlefield and, with hundreds of others, Jane made ready to flee the city. Sixty-three years old, asthmatic, and infirm with gout (a disease she shared with her famous brother), she bundled up her belongings, as she wrote to Ben:

> I brought out what I could pack up in trunks and chests [including] most of the things I had to sell. I wish I could have brought all my effects in the same manner, but the whole of my household furniture . . . I left behind, secured indeed in the house with locks and bars; but those who value not to deprive us of our lives will find a way to break through them if they are permitted.

At the last moment before her departure, Jane received an invitation to stay with the Greene family—distant relations through marriage—at Warwick, Rhode Island, about ten miles south of Providence. The house was jammed with other refugees, and it was an extremely pleasant time of great camaraderie. Late that fall Benjamin came to personally escort his sister to Philadelphia, where she took up residence at her brother's home. Deborah died in December and Jane became mistress of the household where she would remain for over a year.

Little is known of Jane during this period of 1776 and early 1777, though it must have been a happy time for her. It had been twelve years since she had been with Benjamin and now they were in each other's company daily. In that eventful year of 1776, Ben was busy at the Continental Congress and with the discussions leading to the Declaration of Independence. Once this was signed, the Congress appointed Franklin commissioner to France where he would attempt to negotiate a treaty for that country's aid. Though he was past seventy, Benjamin accepted, and in late fall Jane watched with sadness as the armed sloop *Reprisal* carried away her best friend. After nine long years, in September 1785, Ben would finally return to Philadelphia. Although this farewell marked the last time Jane would ever see him, their letters would bridge the distances of the next several years.

Ben wrote promptly, announcing that he had arrived safely in Nantes and was about to undertake the journey to Paris. In a postscript he added, "You can have no conception of the respect with which I am received and treated here by the first people, in my private character; for as yet I have assumed no public one." Perhaps Ben's modesty was unfeigned, but surely he must have realized that he was fast becoming one of the world's most famous men. As a statesman, writer, and scientist he was known in every country, and even the British Loyalists grudgingly held deep admiration for him.

Before his letter could arrive, Jane was writing from Goshen, Pennsylvania, where she and other members of the Franklin clan had fled.

> I was distressed at your leaving us, but as affairs have turned out I have blessed God you were absent, and we have reason to hope you are safe arrived at your port. On hearing the enemy were advancing toward us we thought it necessary to retire to this place, where we hope we are safe and are very comfortable.

They were safe for a while, as Washington's victories at Trenton and Princeton in late 1776 and early 1777 kept the British from Philadelphia. After the American defeat at Brandywine in September, however, General Howe marched on Philadelphia. Jane fled once again, back to Rhode Island, this time to Coventry and the house of one of her granddaughters. She would remain there, with occasional trips to Boston, until 1783.

Throughout the years of the war Jane and Ben continued to write, although because their correspondence was constantly in danger of being intercepted by the British, they were reluctant to engage in any political discussions that might be used to the enemy's advantage. For three years every letter written by Benjamin to his sister was intercepted and destroyed, though it is doubtful that they contained any crucial information. Jane often had to live on rumors, which could be as cruel as they were unfounded. On one occasion, in 1778, she heard that an attempt had been made on his life and that he lay "in a languishing condition" in Paris. She had to await the next ship from France to learn that it was mere propaganda and that, in fact, her brother had just successfully concluded the treaty with France. On the same boat came a letter from Benjamin expressing his concern for her: "I pity my poor old sister to be so harassed and driven about by the enemy; for I feel a little myself the inconvenience of being driven about by my friends." Indeed, Jane and her family were harassed, for the British constantly threatened their location in Rhode Island. Her return letter noted that they had been

> in constant jeopardy since the spring. You will acknowledge this is rather worse than being harried about by one's friends, yet I doubt not but that it is troublesome to you who are so desirous of retirement. I fear you will never be suffered to enjoy it.

Her last statement would prove to be prophetic.

The letters surviving this period show that Jane had slowly worked up the courage to write to her brother in the most personal terms. A fictional anecdote regarding Franklin had been published in the *London Chronicle* and reprinted in American newspapers. It read in part, "A gentleman just returned from France informs us that Dr. Franklin has shaken off entirely the mechanical rust, and commenced the complete courtier." It went on to describe a conversation between Benjamin and the French queen in which he behaved with the most foppish gallantry. Jane responded after reading the article:

> Bless God I now and then hear of your health and glorious achievements in the political way, as well as in the favor of the ladies ("since you have rubbed off the mechanic rust and commenced the complete courtier"), who Jonathan Williams writes me claim from you the tribute of an embrace, and it seems you do not complain of the tax as a very great penance. . . .

Ben replied that "the story you allude to which was in the newspa-

pers, mentioning 'mechanic rust,' etc. is totally without foundation," though he concluded this letter by saying, "I hope, however,
to preserve, while I stay here, the regard you mention of the French
ladies, for their society and conversation, when I have time to enjoy
it, is extremely agreeable." The last written, no doubt, with a bit of a
twinkle in the old eye.

Jane's most direct statement concerning her diminishing timidity
in her relations with Ben came in a letter written to him in July 1779.
In part it referred to a gift he had apparently sent her:

> You, like yourself, do all for me that the most affectionate brother
> can be desired or expected to do. And though I feel myself full of
> gratitude for your generosity, the conclusion of your letter affects me
> more: where you say you wish we may spend our last days together. O
> my brother, if this could be accomplished it would give me more joy
> than anything on this side heaven could possibly do. I feel the want of
> suitable conversation . . . I have but little here. I think I could
> assume more freedom with you now, and convince you of my
> affection for you; for I have had time to reflect and see my error in
> that respect. I suffered my diffidence and the awe of your superiority
> to prevent the familiarity I might have taken with you, and ought, and
> your kindness to me might have convinced me would be acceptable.
> But it is hard overcoming a natural propensity, and diffidence is mine.

Perhaps Benjamin's constant reassurances finally gave her confidence; perhaps in her old age she was looking back over the years
and realizing that she too had lived. Whatever the reasons, her
future letters would be far more confident, written almost as an
equal to her illustrious brother.

In March 1782, Jane's seventieth birthday found her living in
various relatives' homes from Rhode Island to Boston. "I am grown
such a vagrant I can't opine the place I may be in. . . . " she wrote
one of her nieces. She had not heard from her brother in nearly two
years. Although the war had ended with the Battle of Yorktown in
1781, British privateers continued to roam the seas. Apparently all
of Ben's letters had been seized and destroyed by zealous British
censors. As year followed year and no response came from France,
Jane herself began to write fewer letters until they ceased almost
entirely. We know that in 1782 she suffered a period of severe
though undefined illness; nevertheless, by 1783 she was dabbling
once again in her business of millinery sales. Finally, in late 1783
news arrived from Paris that Franklin had effectively brought about

the peace treaty between England and the United States. With it arrived a letter from Ben promising Jane an assured income for life as well as the rental income from a house he owned on Unity Street in Boston. Her return letter in April 1784 was ecstatic.

> I have at length received a letter from you in your own handwriting, after a total silence of three years, in which time part of an old song would sometimes intrude itself into my mind.

> Does he love and yet forsake me?
> For can he forgit me?
> Will he neglect me?

> This was but momentary. At other times I concluded it was reasonable to expect it, and that you might with great propriety, after my teasing you so often, send me the answer that Nehemiah did to Tobiah and Sanballat, who endeavored to obstruct his building the Temple of Jerusalem: "I am doing a great work, so that I cannot come down; why should the work cease, whilst I leave it and come down to you."

> And a great work indeed you have done, God be praised. I hope now you yourself will think you have done enough for the public, and will now put in execution what you have sometimes wished to be permitted to do: sit down and spend the evening with your friends. I am looking round me at Cambridge for a commodious seat for you, not with any great hopes of your coming here, I confess (but wishes), knowing you are accommodated so much to your mind at Philadelphia, and have your children there. I should however expect a share of your correspondence when you have leisure.

In September 1785 Franklin finally arrived back in Philadelphia to a tremendous public welcome. His last letter from France and his first from Philadelphia were written to Jane, describing his departure and arrival. Jane replied on September 23, welcoming him home and saying that she would come immediately to see him if only she could find a traveling companion. Her relatives must all have been predisposed in some way, however, for Jane remained in Boston. Ben surely would have come to her, but he immediately found himself besieged with demands on his time. He was now literally the most famous private citizen in the world, and with fame came separation once again from those he loved. For the next five years he and his sister would be able to visit only through their letters.

That same year Jane renovated the house on Unity Street and moved into it with her last remaining daughter, Jenny, and her husband. It was as Jane described it, "pleasant for light and air." There were no more financial burdens now; her life was looking good, perhaps even promising, though she was well into her seventies. As Benjamin wrote her on January 1, 1786,

> Our good God has brought us old folks, the last survivors of seventeen brothers and sisters, to the beginning of a new year. The measure of health and strength we enjoy at so advanced an age, now near fourscore, is a great blessing. Let us be cheerful and thankful.

Gratitude she certainly felt, and most of it was to her brother who had arranged for her absolute comfort in her later years.

In the flood of adulation that had swept over Franklin upon his return, he had been elected governor of Pennsylvania. Never one to shirk public duty—or to stay out of the limelight—he accepted, and promptly received a letter from his sister. After chatting about a number of things, she concluded, "I rejoice in every honorable mention that is made of you, but I cannot find it in my heart to be pleased at your accepting the government of the state, and therefore have not much congratulated you on it. I fear it will fatigue you too much." This was a good example of what Ben had called years ago, Jane's "miffy temper." He patiently replied that though his gout and gallstones caused him discomfort, "my appetite continues good, and my temper generally cheerful, and strength and activity diminishing indeed, but by slow degrees."

By the following year, Jane had apparently resigned herself to her brother's continued activity, for when news arrived in early 1787 that he had been appointed a delegate to the Federal Convention, which was to frame a new Constitution, she wrote him:

> I wanted to tell you how much pleasure I enjoy in the constant and lively mention of you in the newspapers, which makes you appear to me like a man of twenty-five just setting out for the other eighty years full of great designs for the benefit of mankind, and your own nation in particular; which I hope with the assistance of such a number of wise men as you are connected with in the Convention you will gloriously accomplish, and put a stop to the necessity of dragooning and haltering. They are odious means. I had rather hear of the swords being beat into plowshares and the halters used for cart ropes, if by that means we may be brought to live peaceably with one another.

The Constitution was adopted and signed by September 20, and Ben wrote to Jane that she might see copies of it published in the papers. What he did not mention was that he often had to be carried to the State House in a sedan chair because of his gout. Jane must have heard reports, however, and by 1788 Ben was forced to admit that recurring attacks of one or another of his ailments often kept him confined to his house. But at this time, Jane, too, was often ill.

On Ben's birthday in 1790, Jane wrote to him:

> This day my dear brother completes his eighty-fourth year. You cannot, as old Jacob, say few and evil have they been, except those wherein you have endured such grievous torments latterly. Yours have been filled with innumerable good works, benefits to your fellow creatures, and thankfulness to God; that notwithstanding the distressing circumstances before mentioned, yours must be esteemed a glorious life. Great increase of glory and happiness I hope await you. May God mitigate your pain and continue your patience yet many years. For who that know and love you can bear the thought of surviving you in this gloomy world?

In this letter we find the only reference that either of them made to her looks: "I am as you suppose six years younger than you are, being born on the 27th March 1712, but to appearance in every one's sight as much older."

On March 24 Benjamin wrote to his sister:

> . . . I have been quite free from pain for near three weeks past; and therefore not being obliged to take any laudanum, my appetite has returned, and I have recovered some part of my strength. Thus I continue to live on, while all the friends of my youth have left me, and gone to join the majority. I have, however, the pleasure of continued friendship and conversation with their children and grandchildren. I do not repine at my malady, though a severe one, when I consider how well I am provided with every convenience to palliate it and to make me comfortable under it; and how many more horrible evils the human body is subject to; and what a long life of health I have been blessed with, free from them all.

After some questions about various members of the family, he added a postscript: "It is early in the morning, and I write in bed. The awkward position has occasioned the crooked lines." Over the years Benjamin had written more letters to Jane than to any other single person, and this was his last. On April 17, 1790 he died peacefully and quickly in Philadelphia.

No doubt word of mouth brought the news of his death to Jane before the newspapers or formal letters from the family. Ben's daughter, Sarah Franklin Bache, wrote a week later offering official notice and condolences, but there was no reply from Jane for four months. Only a few months before she had written to Ben, "Who that know and love you can bear the thought of surviving you in this gloomy world?" We can only guess at what her thoughts were now. It is certain that she was surrounded by the remnants of her family for the next few months, and then, there were the newspapers. The extravagant eulogies that poured forth daily in the press must have calmed her grief, for it was clear that the rest of the world held Franklin in the same esteem as did Jane. In September she wrote back to Sarah:

> It is a cordial to my heart to receive such affectionate notice from my dear brother's child. He while living was to me every enjoyment. Whatever other pleasures were, as they mostly took their rise from him, they passed like little streams from a beautiful fountain. . . . To make society agreeable there must be a similarity of circumstances and sentiments, as well as age. I have no such near me; my dear brother supplied all. Every line from him was a pleasure. If I asked questions he did not think proper to inform me on, he would sometimes give me a gentle reproof. At other times he completely passed it over; that I knew was always fitted for the occasion, and all was pleasure. . . . It is, however, very agreeable to me to see there is hardly a newspaper comes out in this town without honorable mention of him; and indeed it is a fund that cannot be exhausted.

The letter closed with the following: "When I sit down to write to you, I think I will try to correct my writing and spelling; but I am grown so infirm and so indolent the task is too arduous. If you can find out what I mean, you must accept it as it is; if not, let me know, and I will get my daughter to write for me."

Jane's health was failing rapidly and the only remaining letters written after this are in her daughter's hand. They discuss only the technicalities of Ben's will, wherein he left Jane sufficient money for several more years of comfortable living. But as to whom she saw or wrote to, or the details of these last years, there is no word.

In January 1794 Jane received notice of the death of her oldest friend, Catherine Greene, with whom she had stayed in Rhode

Island during the war years. It prompted her to write her will, the first paragraph of which read,

> I, Jane Mecom of Boston in the County of Suffolk and Common-wealth of Massachusetts, Widow; being, although weak in body, yet of sound mind and memory; well knowing that the time must arise when I shall be called apon to resign this decaying frame to its parent dust, and my spirit to the God who gave it; do this seventeenth day of February in the year of Our Lord One thousand seven hundred and ninety four, ordain, make and publish this my Last will and testament, in the manner following.

These were the last recorded words of Jane Franklin Mecom. The exact day and manner of her death are not known, nor is the place of her burial. On May 10, 1794, however, the *Columbian Centinel* published the following notice:

> Mrs. Jane Mecom, widow of the late Mr. Edward Mecom of this town, and the only sister of the late Doctor Franklin, in the 83rd year of her age. Her funeral will be this afternoon, precisely at five o'clock, from her late dwelling near the North Church, which her friends, and the friends of the late Dr. Franklin, are requested to attend.

Of course Jane was not Ben's only sister, though she might as well have been, since she was the only one for whom he had an abiding affection. Together they were the greatest of the Franklins, though one was famous and the other obscure. Jane left her mark on history, not only as a mirror in which we see her brother more clearly, but as a woman in her own right.

8

Phillis Wheatley

HER DEATH did not pass unnoticed. "Last Lord's Day," reported Boston's *Independent Chronicle* for December 9, 1784, "died Mrs. Phillis Peters [formerly Phillis Wheatley], aged thirty-one, known to the world by her celebrated miscellaneous poems." It is not known by whom she was mourned. Her husband was in debtor's jail, and her three children were all dead. One who had known her wrote—many years later—that she "was carried to her last resting-place, without one of the friends of her prosperity to follow her, and without a stone to mark her grave."

She died in abject poverty, this poet "known to the world." Many knew *of* her, for indeed she had been celebrated and had had friends of wealth and standing. But that was all before the War of Independence, the war that set her young country free while it established for her the conditions of a terrible bondage.

What the *Independent Chronicle* failed to note, a notice perhaps unnecessary since every literate Bostonian was sure to know, was that Phillis Wheatley had been a slave, the most famous slave in the world. She had been freed midway through the Revolutionary War by the deaths of the last two Wheatleys who had owned her. But that freedom had only consigned her to the prison of poverty.

Later in the month of her death, some anonymous versifier eulogized her in *Boston Magazine*. She was now, "Horatio" wrote, "Free'd from a world of woe, and scene of cares." Indeed, for at her death this freedwoman was working as a domestic in a cheap boardinghouse for blacks, doing the kind of work she had been spared while a slave in the Wheatley household. There, in one of Boston's finer homes, the residence of a respected merchant-tailor, she would only occasionally be allowed, in the words of a Wheatley relative, "to polish a table or dust an apartment or engage in some other trifling occupation." For in the halcyon days before the war, Phillis was encouraged to write and, even as a slave, to visit the fashionable drawing rooms of Boston society where her presence was always welcome.

She had established that honor through her own merits. If she was celebrated in England and the colonies by the age of nineteen, she was known throughout Boston well before that. Boston society had been amazed at the little slave girl who could write and recite such elegant verse.

The Wheatleys, of course, were the first to be astonished. Mrs. Wheatley was looking only for a young slave to help her in her advancing years when she and her husband visited the Boston docks that day in 1761. What had they expected to find? The slaves sold in Boston were, typically, "refuse"—slaves who had been just hardy enough to survive the cruel and arduous journey from Africa to the West Indies and the southern colonies where the strongest and healthiest stock were sold to work in the fields. The rest, most of them young girls and children, were then carried up the coast to Boston where citizens could purchase these "leftovers" at an inexpensive price and use them as household maids and servants.

What the Wheatleys discovered was a poet. They could hardly discern this from her appearance, though—she stood there at auction, newly released from a ship's "tight pack" cargo hold with nothing but a piece of dirty carpet placed around her. She had no name and appeared to be seven or eight years old, for she was shedding her front teeth. Some of the slaves, the Boston newspaper advertisements show, were sold along with cattle and sheep. The Wheatleys purchased only the young girl and took her to their home on King Street in their chaise.

They named her Phillis and gave her to Mary, their eighteen-year-old daughter, for elementary instruction in the English language and in domestic duties. Mary discovered very early that the little girl was quite a mimic, with an amusing capacity to imitate precisely the simple words and sentences that she had said to her. But if she was an entertaining mimic, how well could she learn to read? After all, the girl knew not a word of English when she arrived at the house. She didn't even have a name of her own she could recite!

Mary gave her lessons in the Bible, lessons which were to be as instructive for the teacher as for the student. The little girl learned so rapidly that Mary was at a loss to know what to do with her. When

Mrs. Wheatley visited the lessons, she, too, was surprised beyond belief. It had been only a few months since she had purchased the girl, and Phillis was reading the Bible at a pace that was remarkable. Mr. Wheatley and his son Nathaniel paid little attention to the experiment until one day they saw Phillis, charcoal in hand, scrawling figures on a wall at the back of the house. They supposed she was playing, but were shocked when they looked closely at her marks. Phillis was writing words on the wall!

The slave bought to be a lady's maid was, in fact, a budding prodigy. By the time she had been in the house sixteen months, she was reading even the most difficult portions of the Bible with ease and was writing skillfully. Mary, like most young ladies of the time, knew little more than the Bible, simple geography, and mathematics. The student was too precocious for the mistress. Nathaniel recommended things to read, and books came from neighbors and friends who shared the Wheatleys' befuddled delight.

Phillis was encouraged to read whatever she could. She was given the classics: Horace and Terence—the latter Phillis grew to love especially because he was of African birth—and then Milton and Pope and Gray. Phillis began to read with Mary books that the mistress thought she herself would never read. And she was writing in a fashion that Mary could have profited from through imitation. By early adolescence, Phillis was corresponding with many notables in Boston, and beyond. Mrs. Wheatley was especially proud that she even wrote a letter to an Indian minister in London!

With Phillis fluent in English, the Wheatleys were curious to see if the little girl could explain her startling development. Where, indeed, had she come from? What had life been like there? Who were her parents? Did she remember anything?

The Wheatleys wouldn't have known that her African heritage had perhaps something to do with her remarkable abilities. All she could remember of her past was an image of her mother pouring water on the land before the rising sun, honoring the new day by the rite. The ritual would have been a Moslem one, and in that case Phillis would have known the Arabic language. Such experience would partially account for her remarkable abilities with language and indeed, her developing devout religious sensibilities.

For the Wheatleys, however, Phillis's recollection indicated that her mother had been a pagan. Her pouring water to greet the rising sun was the act of a heathen religion. Many had already told Phillis she was fortunate, because in coming to America she was coming to a land of Christians, people whom the glorious God would save from their sins, as the Bible told. She was especially fortunate because, as she knew from her Bible, the black children of Cain were marked for perdition.

She would be saved by giving herself up to that God. She wrote in her Bible in prayer: "Oh my Gracious Preserver! . . Tho conceived in Sin & brot forth in iniquity yet thy infinite wisdom can bring a clean thing out of an unclean, a vessel of Honor filled for Thy glory—grant me to live a life of gratitude to Thee for the innumerable benefits—O Lord my God! Instruct my ignorance and enlighten my darkness."

She would spend her brief life writing poems, the most famed in the colony, celebrating her faith in both the God who had saved her and in the white culture that, she believed, had given her the opportunity to be saved. In coming to America, she knew she had experienced something similar to that experienced by the founding Puritans of New England. She told a slave friend she had undergone a "saving change."

That change, the "high calling," as she named it, was confirmed for her in her adolescence when she was baptized in the Old South Meetinghouse. Consigned to a seat with other slaves in the gallery of the church, she was accepted there as "Phillis, servant to Mr. Wheatley." If the ceremony was simple, Phillis did not respond in a simple manner. She was exceptionally devout, and in her mind her identity as both an African and an American was infused with a special religiosity. She was, above all, a Christian.

If blacks were to be marked by their color to be outside God's favor, she rebelled against the idea, for as she later wrote, " 'Twas mercy brought me from my Pagan land,/Taught my benighted soul to understand/That there's a God, and there's a Savior too." She responded to the popular idea that the color black was "a diabolic dye" by admonishing Christians to remember that "Negroes, black as Cain,/May be refin'd, and join the angelic train."

She would hold herself up as an example of the possibilities of refinement at a time when it was conventional folk wisdom to believe that black skins contained blackened souls bound for everlasting damnation. Later at the height of her fame, she would support the return of black Christians to Africa for evangelical purposes. Her frail condition and her need to aid a dying mistress prevented her from a fuller commitment, but she wrote a sponsor of the idea that "What I can do in influencing my Christian friends and acquaintances, to promote this laudable design, shall not be found wanting." Africa, she thought, suffered from "spiritual famine," and she was happy to foresee "at distant time the thick cloud of ignorance dispersing from the face of my benighted country."

It was with such ideas that Phillis first began to write the poetry that was to earn her international fame. One early poem, written when she was barely fifteen, was addressed to university students in nearby Cambridge, offering to advise these fledglings in the ways of the world from the vantage of her own experience. She had left, she wrote, "my native shore/The land of Errors, and *Egyptian* gloom," guided from "those dark abodes" by God. She warned the students against "sin, that baneful evil to the soul."

Phillis's special status as a black Christian was complicated by her status as an extraordinary slave. She was conscious of her darkness in both a religious and racial sense. Certainly she was special in the Wheatley household. She had only light duties, and she could visit the most distinguished people in Boston to recite her poems. She was allowed to keep beside her bed a light and a pen and stationery so that she might record those moments when words and images came to her in the night and she transformed them into poems. Sometimes she would be allowed the privilege of keeping a fire going all night in her room, so that she could be warm when she stayed up late to write.

In this special position, she was permitted to do things other slaves surely were not allowed to do. At the same time, she was a slave. This meant that even as she was being honored, she maintained a sense of both genuine modesty and sharp-witted prudence. Always when visiting, a relative of the Wheatleys would later recall, Phillis "declined the seat offered at their board, and, requesting that a side-table might be laid for her, dined modestly apart from the rest of the company."

If she thus excluded herself from the full company of whites, she was doubly alienated, for she was not allowed by the Wheatleys the full company of blacks. This was pointed out to her daily by the special privileges which marked her off from the other servants. Mrs. Wheatley was especially possessive: the slave was for her a rare prize. On occasion this fact would become graphically clear to Phillis. One damp, cold day, when Phillis was visiting friends of the Wheatley family at some distance from King Street, Prince, the black slave who drove the carriage, called for her at Mrs. Wheatley's bidding. He took Phillis home, and during the ride she decided she would sit on top with him. When they arrived at King Street, the lady grew wrathful: "Do but look at the saucy varlet, if he hasn't the impudence to sit upon the same seat as my Phillis," she cried. The rebuke was directed at Prince, but implicitly, Phillis must have known, to herself as well.

With a life marked by such ambiguity, Phillis devoted herself fully to her writing. The reward was immediate recognition since she was such a rarity. It had been more than a century since the colony had seen such a fine female poet. Phillis's predecessor, Ann Bradstreet, was still popular with Boston readers and was noted, like Phillis, for her religious sentiments.

But never before had there appeared a black woman poet like Phillis. Technically the honor would go to Lucy Terry, a black slave from Deerfield, far in the interior of the colony, who had written in 1746 of an Indian raid on that village. Lucy Terry, who was to become famous as an orator, had written in a rough verse and language hardly suited to please a genteel audience of how "Eunice Allen see the Indians comeing/And hoped to save herself by running/And had not her petticoats stopt her/The awful creatures had not cotched her/And tommyhawked her on the head/And left her on the ground for dead."

Phillis's sensibility was more finely developed. In 1770 she earned fame throughout the colonies and in England with an ode on the death of the famous religious leader George Whitefield. This choice of subject earned her the sponsorship of Countess Huntingdon in England, Whitefield's patroness, who had greatly appreciated the poem.

The choice of subject is also emblematic of the limitations she placed upon herself as a poet. The year 1770 was extremely significant, especially to those inhabiting Phillis's immediate surroundings. It was the year of the Boston Massacre, an event which took place so close to the Wheatley home that she might have even heard the musket blasts. "All the bells in town were ringing," one eyewitness reported, so Phillis must have heard them. The event might have had special significance for her since one of its victims was Crispus Attucks, a slave like herself, though he was a runaway.

But she did not write about the massacre, choosing instead an English religious leader she had undoubtedly heard preaching at one time on the Boston Common. If her passions were moved by politics, she kept them pretty much in check, avoiding controversy when she could.

It was not that she lacked patriotism; rather, she chose other topics since taking sides could compromise her position as a slave. She ventured only occasionally in those years into the realm of

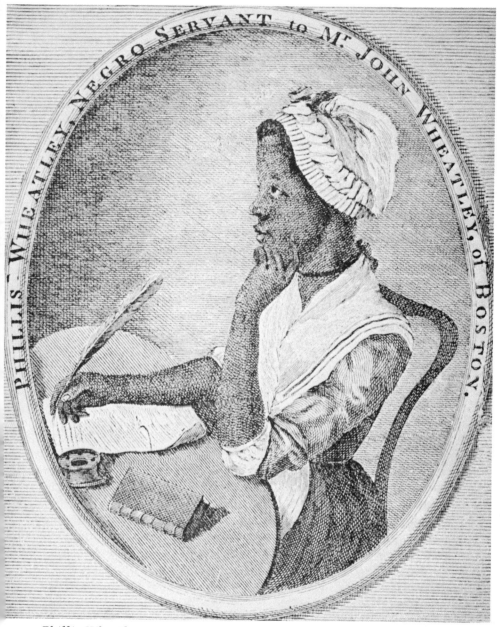

Phillis Wheatley
Courtesy, Historical Pictures Service, Chicago

political ideas, as when she wrote, two years before the massacre, a poem praising King George III on his repeal of the Stamp Act. She told the king, "A monarch's smile can set his subjects free." Her ideas at the time were the ideas of the Patriots who, like her master, sought self-determination without, if it could be prevented, offending the British Crown.

That Phillis felt the issues not "politically" but personally is evident from a poem she wrote in 1772. It was addressed to Lord Dartmouth, an important figure to the colonists, for he had been instrumental in the passage of the repeal and was now the king's secretary of state to the colonies. He was a special person to Phillis, for like Whitefield he was an intimate of Lady Huntingdon's religious circle, a group she felt emotionally close to. In praising Dartmouth's appointment and his virtues, she also stated as eloquently as she ever would, her own necessary attachment to the American cause.

Through the poem she expressed a special "love of Freedom," for she had been "snatched from Africa's fancied happy seat," causing, she knew, "excruciating" pain and sorrow for her parents. She concluded:

Such, such my case. And can I then but pray
Others may never feel tyrranic sway?

The poem, the most specific statement of her own situation as an African and slave as she was ever to confess, was as well a barely implicit warning to the parent England that should it continue its tyranny, England would itself experience great trauma and grief in the loss of its child. In her burgeoning fame, she could hardly have known then that though she was correct that England would suffer greatly, the war would also mean for her intense anguish and even death.

But now in 1773, not yet twenty years old, she was poised upon a great moment—her voyage to England. Mrs. Wheatley had visited there a year earlier and had partially prepared for Phillis's trip by bringing to Lord Dartmouth her poem to him. Phillis was going primarily for her health, for doctors thought that in her asthmatic condition a spring sail across the Atlantic would do her much good. So she went with Nathaniel who was traveling to England for business.

She went well-prepared to be received as the most eminent poet in the colonies, even though that status was emphasized remarkably by her being a slave. On her voyage she carried a letter from her master and messages from some of the most honored men in Boston, including the governor and John Hancock, testifying to her abilities to write poetry. The famous men of Boston wrote that the girl who had been an "uncultivated barbarian from Africa . . . has been examined by some of the best Judges, and is thought qualified" to write verse.

She was going to be received by British nobility, was expecting even to meet the king, but her condition as a slave stayed with her. The Wheatleys wished, Phillis's mistress wrote Lady Huntingdon, that even though their charge had been given money to buy clothes, "she should be dress'd plain. . . . "

The stay in England marked the publication of her first volume of verse, the first ever by a black woman. Major periodicals in London reviewed the volume, which made her the best known colonial poet. Some called her poems "merely imitative" and "of no astonishing powers of genius," while others both praised her writing and expressed outrage that she should still be a slave. Apparently word of her success reached France, for the next year Voltaire praised Phillis's writing in a letter to a friend.

Phillis herself was excited about the publication and worked to promote the sale of the volume, which she entitled *Poems on Various Subjects, Religious and Moral.* Altogether she was surprised at her reception. Writing later to a slave friend, Obour Tanner, at Newport, Rhode Island, she said, "The friends I found there among the Nobility and Gentry, Their benevolent conduct toward me, the unexpected and unmerited civility and Complaisance with which I was treated by all, fills me with astonishment, I can scarcely realize it. . . . "

But there were qualifications to the great victory. She arrived in London late in the season, and thus missed her invited audience with King George at St. James, for the court had already moved from London for the summer season. It is even unlikely that she saw her patroness, Lady Huntingdon, for in a letter written to the lady just before she was called back to America by the illness of Mrs. Wheatley, Phillis expressed regret that she had not yet seen "my friend." The criticism of her poetry had bothered her as well, for in the same letter she thanked the countess for her patronage which softened, and she referred feistily to "the severe trials of Uppity criticism." Her departing gift from the Lord Mayor of London would prove an omen for the times to come—a prized copy of one of her favorites, Milton's *Paradise Lost.*

Upon returning to America, she found Mrs. Wheatley very ill. Having been treated somewhat like a daughter, Phillis felt like a family member, and many told her how the ailing Mrs. Wheatley had missed her greatly. Phillis had sent a copy of an engraving of herself which had appeared in her volume of poems, and Mrs. Wheatley had placed it prominently over the fireplace. One day, the grandniece of the lady later recalled, the woman stared at the engraving and exclaimed: "See! Look at my Phillis! Does she not seem as though she would speak to me!"

The lady died in March 1774, Phillis having spent much of her time since her return from London tending to her needs. She wrote to Obour: "I have lately met with a great trial in the Death of my mistress; let us imagine the loss of a Parent, Sister or Brother, the tenderness of all these were united in her—I was a poor little outcast & Stranger when she took me in . . . I was treated more like a child than a servant."

Mrs. Wheatley's death was to presage Phillis's increasing difficulties in Boston. If she was excited in early May, writing in a letter to Obour that ships from England had brought 300 more of her volumes to sell in Boston, she must have been forlorn by June 1, for on that day began the blockade of Boston Harbor. For a poet who had always downplayed political events in her poetry, politics was now severely interfering with her career (and, importantly for her pride, with the receipt of money for sales of her volume, part of which she could keep for herself). The blockade meant no more deliveries from England. Ironically, one of the notable men of Boston who had vouched for her ability to write—John Hancock— was the mastermind of the Boston Tea Party the preceding December, the act which precipitated the retaliatory blockade.

With the war imminent, Mrs. Wheatley dead, and other family members and friends increasingly occupied by the developments, Phillis was slowly to discover that her tenure as America's most popular public poet was in jeopardy. If she was to continue as a public poet, one whose occasional verse would celebrate virtues and mourn the deaths of the great, she would now have to ready herself to respond to that most extremely public of events—war. In reality, only one great moment of recognition remained.

She had written a poem to General Washington in October 1775, to celebrate his appointment as commander in chief of the armies of

North America. The poem showed perhaps some prescience on her part, for in one of the versions that has been published she pictured Washington as "First in Peace," thus looking forward both to the successful completion of the war and Washington's postwar preeminence. The commander was both amused and pleased by the poem but did not want to publish it because, as he wrote to his secretary, he was afraid such publication would "be considered rather as a mark of my own vanity, than as a compliment to her."

It is likely that at first the general didn't even know of Phillis's reputation as a slave poet, for he referred to her as "Mrs. or Miss Phillis Wheatley" to his secretary. If he knew she were a slave, he, a slaveholder himself, would never have experienced the polite confusion over whether Phillis was a "Mrs. or Miss." But he soon discovered her identity, for in a letter four months later addressed to "Miss Phillis," Washington praised her poem as a "new instance of your genius" and told her "If you should ever come to Cambridge, I shall be happy to see a person so favored by the Muses, and to whom Nature has been so beneficent in her dispensations."

The visit was an easy one for Phillis to make. Although she had resided with the Wheatleys in Providence a year earlier, following their evacuation from British-occupied Boston, she was now living with Wheatley relatives in Chelsea, close to the captured city and Cambridge. She visited Washington in March and, despite the fact that the commander must have been quite busy assembling an army, she received during her half-hour stay, in the words of one of the general's staff, "the most polite attention of the Commander-in-Chief."

Hopefully, she gloried in her visit, for Washington was the last public figure to honor her in her lifetime. Soon—with the war raging—she was to receive notice from no one.

Her talents were simply not geared for the requirements of poetry in time of war, an ironic fact given the publication of her poem to Washington in the *Pennsylvania Magazine*—the journal edited by the radical pamphleteer Tom Paine. The war called for ringing prose and straightforward calls to arms to stir a disinterested public—the kind of writing that Paine would continue to produce. The slave poet's ornate diction and classical meter and allusions hardly stirred the heart to fight, and that was the obligation of the time.

As she was to discover, her poems had lost their readers, who made up the elite of society. Those of them who took up the

Patriots' cause were too busy to read of elevated matters. Her other earlier readers were Loyalists who—having fled on account of the war to Canada or England—were quite literally lost to her.

Again she tried. A year after her poem to Washington, she responded to the war with a poem on the capture of the American Major General Charles Lee by British dragoons in New Jersey. Though the thoughts behind the poem were combative enough for any reader, the style and diction were hardly suitable for a public caught up in war. In the poem she had Lee address the British in a manner that is denied its heat by the cool form and language of the speaker:

> What various causes to the field invite!
> For plunder *you,* and we for freedom fight.
> Her cause divine with generous ardor fires,
> And every bosom glows as she inspires!
> Already, thousands of your troops are fled
> To the Drear mansions of the silent dead:
> Columbia too, beholds with streaming eyes
> Her heroes fall—'tis freedom's sacrifice!

It was to be a long time before she would publish another poem. She fell into silence, perhaps because she knew how out of step she was. Even her choice of subject for her poetry seemed ill-conceived, for Major General Lee, though a popular figure when she published her poem, was later to enter into a treasonous relationship with the British. Her personal life became extremely chaotic, and even her faithful correspondence with her slave friend Obour Tanner lapsed until 1778.

When she finally began writing to her friend again, the tone of her remarks as much as the content indicated her saddened state: "The vast variety of scenes that have passed before us these 3 years past will to a reasonable mind serve to convince us of the uncertain duration of all things temporal." She thought that "the proper result of such a consideration is an ardent desire of & preparation for a state of enjoyments which are more suitable for the immortal mind."

Phillis had only a half-hour to ready this letter to Obour, for during the war, mail service was announced infrequently and suddenly. Perhaps because of the haste she failed to mention what Obour could have learned earlier through informal means—that Phillis was now both free and a wife. Obour must have been shocked at her friend's despondency and apparent longing for death.

While the young country was fighting for its freedom, Phillis was handed her liberty rather by default. Both her old master and Mary, who had taught her how to read and write, died in 1778. Nathaniel, who had taken her on her great trip to England, was the immediate family's lone survivor, but he was now in England, apparently siding with the Loyalists.

She had been freed, but freed into a state of uncertainty in a nation whose war mirrored her own chaos. If she were masterless, she had no skills or abilities or even physical strength to market and was thus still enslaved. She acted to resolve her dilemma on April 1 by marrying John Peters whom Phillis had met four years earlier and whom she thought, as she wrote to Obour at the time, "a complaisant and agreeable young man."

Others had different reactions to him. Obour told her mistress that she thought "poor Phillis let herself down by marrying," and a Wheatley relative found him "disagreeable," a man of "improper conduct." He had had a varied career as a free black, trying his hand at being a baker, a barber, a lawyer, and even a doctor. Whether he was admirably inventive in a time when blacks had few formal opportunities or was merely an opportunist and charlatan, the opinion of many whites who knew him was that he was "shiftless." But that epithet was frequently applied to blacks, especially to an uncommonly proud black like Peters who, in the words of a Wheatley relative, "quite acted out 'the gentleman,' " sporting wig and cane.

No doubt Phillis was attracted to him, not only because he was handsome, but also because he was, like herself, highly articulate. She would have had few black suitors of equal abilities, very few who, like Peters, had at one time "pleaded the cause of his brethren, the Africans, before the tribunals of the State." But if her new husband had been successful at one time, his career during the war was to prove an utter failure. The chaotic times made it impossible for him to practice a trade or profession with any regularity, and his inability or refusal to work at menial labor meant the Peters family was to live in poverty.

Times were not merely bad; they were horrid. Goods were scarce and inflation ran rampant throughout the colonies. The Peters retreated to Wilmington in the interior, but undoubtedly even the inland areas were suffering like the capital city. There the Peters heard of and experienced the same kind of hardships that they had heard of and experienced in Boston—a man selling a cow for forty dollars and paying the same sum for a goose; another man buying a cord of wood for over a thousand dollars; a woman paying fifty dollars for a quarter of barely edible mutton.

Unable to survive in Wilmington, her first child already dead in infancy, Phillis left her husband and returned to the Wheatley family after a year, taking up residence with a niece of Mrs. Wheatley who conducted a day school in her war-battered house in Boston. She wrote again to Obour in May 1779, quiet about her difficulties, hoping only that "our correspondence will revive—and revive in better times."

Once more she turned her hand to poetry, hoping that if she could sell her verse, the money would allow John and her to live together again. She advertised in October 1779, the sale by subscription of a volume of thirty-three poems and thirteen letters, her first production as "Phillis Peters," though readers would have recognized the former slave by her self-description in the advertisement: "A *female* African, whose lot it was to fall into the hands of a *generous* master and *great* benefactor."

All the benefactors were gone now, and nobody bought the volume. Undoubtedly it was too precious in price and perhaps appearance for a country at war—a "neatly Bound and Lettered" copy selling for twelve pounds, another "sew'd in blue paper" being offered at nine pounds.

Between her unsuccessful attempt at selling her poems and the war's end, Phillis worked in the day school, and after that in a common Negro boardinghouse, earning her own subsistence by cleaning. She gave birth to another child, and this one also died in infancy. She wrote only rarely but celebrated the war's end when it came. "From every tongue celestial Peace resounds," she wrote, and she pictured the darkness of war being driven away by the brightness of peace:

So freedom comes array'd with Charms divine
And in her Train Commerce and Plenty shine.

When the poem finally appeared in print in 1784, her husband had been almost a year in debtor's jail, and she had been dead several days—a freedwoman in bondage. With her died her third child.

PART III

Those Dashing Ladies of the Opposition

9

Rebecca Franks

SHORTLY AFTER THE CLOSE of the War of 1812, the American General Winfield Scott embarked on a European tour. With him he carried letters of introduction to various notables which had been provided by prominent members of New York and Philadelphia society. Approaching the city of Bath, England, Scott sent ahead a letter which recommended him to a certain Lady Johnson, wife of the Baronet Sir Henry Johnson, a senior general in the British army. In the Revolutionary War, Johnson had been a colonel under the command of Clinton at New York, where he had met and married the former Rebecca Franks, daughter of a wealthy Jewish merchant of Philadelphia.

It was now 1816 and due to years of bad health, Lady Johnson had become prematurely old, even ghostly in her appearance, but her eyes were still bright and her wits intact. As Rebecca Franks she had been one of the reigning belles of Philadelphia, renowned for her beauty, her eccentricity and acid humor, and her extreme and outspoken Loyalist sympathies. Now Sir Henry ushered General Scott into the presence of his imperious wife who had been rolled out in an easy chair to greet him. "Is this the young rebel?" were her first words. "My dear, it is your countryman!" Sir Henry quickly added, fearing that Scott might take offense. Scott politely dodged the accusation as best he could, but the woman followed it up with specific references to several battles during the recent war in which Scott had been victorious.

The atmosphere was becoming somewhat strained when suddenly Lady Johnson reached for Scott's hand and pulled him into a chair beside her. "I have gloried in my rebel countrymen!" she exclaimed with great emotion. "Would to God I, too, had been a

Patriot." The party sat in stunned silence a moment. Finally, Sir Henry interposed that his wife should remember where her current loyalties lay. But Lady Johnson looked up at her husband and said, "I do not; I have never regretted my marriage. No woman was ever blessed with a kinder, a better husband; but I ought to have been a Patriot before marriage."

It is impossible to tell whether this was only the momentary sentiment of an old woman, or if her attitudes had really changed. Even as a mere emotional outburst, however, it indicates a person somewhat different from the Rebecca Franks of thirty-five years before.

In 1740 two young brothers, David and Moses Franks, moved from New York to Philadelphia. Their father, Jacob Franks, had come to America from London and had established himself as a successful businessman. Now his sons were off to make their own fortunes.

Accompanying David and Moses was Nathan Levy, their mother's nephew and an established merchant seventeen years David's senior. Nathan became the Franks brothers' mentor in mercantile affairs, and by 1745 the firm of Levy and Franks was one of the most prosperous in Philadelphia. By 1750 the firm owned three large ships, its own wharves and warehouses in Philadelphia, and had established Moses as its agent in London. Iron, agricultural exports, and timber were sent to England in return for manufactured goods. At least once a year a huge cargo of East Indian goods consigned to Levy and Franks was landed on the Philadelphia wharves. In August 1752 one of the firm's most interesting imports arrived on their ship, the *Myrtilla*—the Liberty Bell which had been ordered for the State House on the occasion of the fiftieth anniversary of Penn's Charter of Liberties for Pennsylvania.

Perhaps the most interesting aspect of the Frankses' rise in the economic world of the colonies is the fact that they were Jews. Beginning in 1654 most of the Jews who emigrated to America were fleeing various forms of racial and religious oppression. Many others came in search of new opportunities. Though they were all subject to the British Crown, they were not considered citizens, and prior to 1740 special laws forbade Jews to vote, to hold public office, or to own property. In 1740, however, the Naturalization Act of George II permitted Jews to gain citizenship by swearing allegiance to the Crown on the Old Testament only, and the former oath that required belief in a Christian God was omitted.

The Frankses and the Levys had migrated from London and were British citizens. They were, therefore, unaffected by the Naturalization Act and any legal restrictions imposed on other immigrant Jews.

By the 1740s David Franks had become democratically ambivalent in his support of both Christian and Jewish affairs. Throughout his life he continued his annual contributions to the Shearith Israel congregation in New York and even attended services there on occasion, but he was also a member of two very exclusive, and decidedly Christian, clubs—the Library Company of Philadelphia and the Mount Regale Fishing Company. It was no secret that David Franks was Jewish, and apparently he was well accepted in the community.

When the war came, however, the fact that he was a Jew, added to his Loyalist sympathies, thrust him back into the old pattern of social discrimination. If he was not convinced that an independent United States was desirable, he was a loyal and productive member of the Philadelphia community and, as such, deserved better treatment than he got. Despite the general air of tolerance in colonial America, political turmoil and economic upsets would cause the old biases to resurface from time to time.

In 1743 David Franks married Margaret Evans, daughter of Peter Evans, Philadelphia's Registrar of Wills. The Evans family was Episcopalian, and though they were not bothered by the fact that David was a Jew, the Franks family took a dim view of the match. David's sister Phila had eloped with the scion of a prominent New York Episcopalian family a year before and was immediately baptized a Christian. David's mother went to her grave thoroughly convinced that she had been a failure as a Jewish mother, since David's four children, including Rebecca, were baptized at Christ Church and raised as Episcopalians.

Like most girls of her time and social position, Rebecca began her public life about the age of fifteen, or sixteen, at the outbreak of the Revolutionary War. From 1776 until her marriage in 1782, she would pursue the active social life that brought her fame. Philadelphia was the center of social life in the colonies, and through Rebecca Franks we can get a picture of what that life was like. The story unfolds in an atmosphere of shifting and uncertain political loyalties that was common not only in most American cities and towns, but also within individual families. The Franks family characterizes this situation perfectly, and some knowledge of their activities before and during the war will set the stage for the story of Rebecca's peculiar career as a society belle in wartime.

In the years prior to the war, David Franks's attitudes were very much like those of other leading Americans—the colonies should remain under the general rule of English law and institutions, though they should have more autonomous control of their own internal affairs. However, when the final decision to pursue open rebellion came, David Franks's ostensible neutrality, his interests in continuing business with the British, and his numerous friends among the British aristocracy would place him in an uncomfortable position notably different from that of most other Jews and many of his former associates. Franks was probably not quite the rabid Loyalist that history has often accused him of being. His daughter Rebecca, on the other hand, would prove to be more decided in her loyalties.

The Patriot presence in Philadelphia had been obvious ever since the First Continental Congress in August 1774. In late winter 1775, the war had begun in earnest and Continental troops were very much in evidence in that city. Washington's army and the various militias that served under his command were a ragged lot—they had no uniforms and carried their own weapons for the most part. When Washington first marched through Philadelphia, the only common identification for his troops was a sprig of green stuck into each of the men's caps. On the other hand, several of the officers were of the gentry and were decked out resplendently in uniforms of their own purchase, seated astride fine horses. If they didn't quite cut the figure of the well-provisioned and elegantly accoutered British soldier, they were equally as charming and the young ladies of Philadelphia welcomed them with open arms.

Although only sixteen years old, Rebecca was already well-known in the drawing rooms and ballrooms of the town. Within a few years she and her friend—and sometimes rival—Peggy Shippen would become the reigning socialites. Peggy, the daughter of a leading attorney, would marry Benedict Arnold in 1779, shortly before he went over to the British side. In 1775, however, Arnold was simply one of a number of gallant young officers who, along with other prospective notables such as Jack Steward and Charles Lee, was courting the favors of the belles of Philadelphia.

Rebecca Franks was described as a beauty very much in the fashionable style of the day—dark haired with pale skin, high cheekbones, a long thin nose, long graceful neck, and an ample bosom barely constrained by low-cut dresses. She was selfish, vain, and given wholly to her own pleasures, though she was also a formidable opponent in the battle of wits that was the favorite pastime of Philadelphia's privileged class. Even her critics grudgingly admired her for her obvious intelligence and the air of complete independence with which she moved through the world. Thoroughly oblivious to the problems of others, however, she was rapidly becoming a millstone around her father's neck. And he did not need her to add to his troubles.

Because of his excellent service during the French and Indian War, David Franks received the commission of supplying British troops through the London firm of his brother, Moses. At first this was acceptable to even the most patriotic Americans since it was clear that someone would have to provision the British, and the profits might as well go to a colonial rather than to a British agent. By late winter 1775, however, Franks's duties increased and complicated his political position in the community.

In the eighteenth century it was common practice for armies to pay for the upkeep of their own men who had been captured by the enemy. General Howe, commandant of the British force, decided that it would be expedient if Franks would supply the British prisoners. At the same time, Congress appointed Franks to provide for the American prisoners of war, and by 1777 he had become the subordinate to the commissary general of prisoners, responsible for the welfare of both the British and the Americans.

In the eyes of all, this was perfectly legitimate business, but, of course, it was too massive a task for any one man or firm. Therefore, Franks let out much of this provisioning to subcontractors, each of whom supplied his own capital and expected to be reimbursed in cash. In theory, Franks and his agents supplied both the British and the Americans with goods paid for with actual specie. Franks was to collect, in specie, from the Congress and the British command what was due him for his goods. He would then pay his subcontractors and retain his profit.

With Continental currency rapidly depreciating in value, and pounds sterling and Spanish gold in short supply in the colonies, both the Congress and the British took a rather cavalier attitude toward Franks's legitimate demands for payment. Soon Franks was in trouble with his subcontractors on the one hand for lack of money, and with the British and Americans on the other, because the subcontractors were refusing to deliver provisions without payment. Franks appealed to Congress that he be allowed to go to British headquarters in New York to adjust his claims there. As early as 1776, he and his clerk were permitted to go on the condition that they "give their promise not to give any intelligence to the enemy, and that they will return to this city." But the trip was a failure, and as the provisioning system began to fall apart, Franks became the scapegoat. Good Patriots openly denounced the "Jew Merchant" for attempting to perform the very services with which he had been charged by Congress. To make things worse, his daughter was becoming the Loyalist darling of Philadelphia.

After the American defeat at Brandywine in 1777, General Howe and his army occupied Philadelphia. The Congress fled to York, Pennsylvania, and General Washington went into winter camp at Valley Forge—only a short distance from Philadelphia. Suddenly the relaxed and somewhat shabby American military presence was replaced by the highly regimented, scarlet-coated formality of the British. Most outspoken Patriots left town but, as is generally the case, much of the population was either apolitical or had avoided discussing political sympathies in public. With little fear of personal recriminations, life in Philadelphia went on much as before.

The young ladies of fashion and high society had even less to fear. Whatever their personal sympathies, and however loudly they might voice them, they were in such demand for all the gay affairs of the town that they were shown a great deal of tolerance. It was this way under both the British and American occupations of the city—where others might be imprisoned or tarred and feathered for expressing views contrary to the ones of those currently in power, the ladies of the upper classes enjoyed almost complete freedom of speech. As Howe and his men discovered that this old Quaker city was not quite as staid as they had imagined, a season of revelry began such as Philadelphia had never seen, producing a gaiety which would ultimately lead to Howe's downfall. For their part the belles of Philadelphia welcomed the British with as much enthusiasm as they had the Americans two years before. Not the least of these was Rebecca Franks, whose proclivity for grand style and elegance immediately attracted her to the British garrison.

Sometime in 1778, a book of rhymes was circulated in Philadelphia that became an instant success with both Loyalists and the British. *The Times—A Poem by Camilo Querio—Poet Laureate of the Congress* contained a number of vicious attacks such as this one on George Washington:

Was it ambition, vanity, or spite
That prompted thee with Congress to unite?
Or did all three within thy bosom roll?
Thou heart of a hero, with a traitor's soul.

It was widely assumed that Rebecca was in fact the celebrated Camilo Querio and had had the booklet published secretly at her own expense. Whether it was true or not, her uncharacteristic silence on the issue was enough to confirm the belief, and the British gloated over having such a lovely American-born Loyalist in their midst. An angry Congress viewed all of this from afar, keeping in mind whose daughter she was.

Throughout the severe winter of 1778, a few miles to the west at Valley Forge, Washington's army was experiencing heavy loss of life from disease, exposure, and starvation. In Philadelphia, however, and especially in Loyalist circles, the gaiety was reaching a fever pitch. In a letter to Mrs. William Paca, Rebecca wrote:

> You can have no idea of the life of continued amusement I live in. I can scarce have a moment to myself. I have stole this while everybody is retired to dress for dinner. I am but just come from under Mr. J. Black's hands and most elegantly am I dressed for a ball this evening at Smith's where we have one every Thursday. You would not know the room 'tis so much improved.
>
> [I am at] no loss for partners, even I am engaged to seven different gentlemen for you must know 'tis a fixed rule never to dance but two dances at a time with the same person. Oh how I wish Mr. P. wou'd let you come in for a week or two—tell him I'll answer for your being let to return. I know you are as fond of a gay life as myself—you'd have an opportunity of rakeing as much as you choose either at plays, balls, concerts or assemblies. I've been but three evenings alone since we moved to town. I begin now to be almost tired.

The social life of Philadelphia made it so easy to forget the rebellious colonials that General Howe and his staff spent most of the winter enjoying themselves. Huge quantities of old wines were consumed, great banquets were a biweekly, if not nightly, affair, and since their presence was in constant demand at the functions of the elite, there was little time for the British command to conduct a war. By early spring it had become clear to the king and Parliament in London that Howe had few if any plans for the next campaign, and he was recalled to explain his behavior. Sir Henry Clinton was to assume command of the British forces in America.

In the spirit of so pleasant a winter, however, the British officers felt that one last entertainment should be held. General Howe had been very popular, and despite the fact that he was facing certain reprimand, it was generally agreed that he should depart in grand style. Accordingly, an elaborate fete was planned—the famous, or if you were a Patriot, infamous—Meschianza, which Howe's critics called his triumph upon leaving America unconquered.

The Meschianza was perhaps one of the most extravagant and opulent festivities in American history, made even more bizarre by the fact that it took place in what was technically a fortified camp in the midst of war. Meschianza comes from the Italian word for a mixture or medley, and it was certainly that—it must rank as one of the great, if frivolous, examples of eighteenth-century eclecticism. At the very center of the event stood Rebecca Franks.

The affair was planned for May 18, 1778, and weeks of preparation went into it. Major John André took charge of most of the planning. He was an excellent artist, a poet of some minor talents and, in general, a man of widely varied skills. In early April he set to work designing, constructing, and painting everything—from the invitations to the ladies' hats to the scenery for the theatricals.

On the appointed day at three o'clock in the afternoon, the party assembled at Knight's Wharf on the Delaware River. Among the company were more than fifty young women of Philadelphia society, many of whom, it must be noted, were daughters of known Patriot families. At the wharf the party was received by a vast number of barges, boats, and galleys, variously decorated with the flags of other nations and states. Ironically, the stars and stripes also flew from one of the masts. As the so-called regatta sailed down the river, military bands played from the larger craft while salvos of cannon fire boomed from the 300 British ships lying at anchor in the harbor.

A few miles downstream the fleet arrived at Walnut Grove, a country estate. Upon disembarking, the company moved up a narrow avenue which opened onto a lawn where an amazing scene had been set. The first entertainment was to be a tournament conducted according to the rules of ancient chivalry.

On either side of the field rose two pavilions of medieval design, fronted by rows of benches arranged like bleachers. Each pavilion bore the standard of one of the two groups of combatants who would take part in the tourney—on the left the Knights of the Blended Rose, and on the right the Knights of the Burning Mountain.

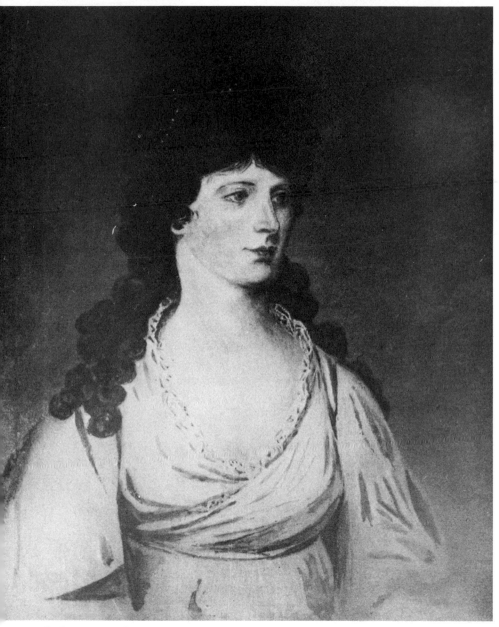

Rebecca Franks
Courtesy, American Jewish Historical Society

A herald, accompanied by two trumpeters, rode out onto the field and bellowed his challenge:

> The Knights of the Blended Rose, by me their herald, proclaim and assert that the ladies of the Blended Rose excel in wit, beauty, and every other accomplishment over all other ladies in the world, and if any knight or knights shall be so hardy to deny this, they are determined to support their assertion by deed of arms, agreeable to the laws of ancient chivalry.

A moment later, the crowd parted on the other side of the field and another herald in orange and black rode forward to assure the ladies of the Burning Mountain that their claims to wit, beauty, and charm would be vindicated by the knights whose colors they wore, "against the false and vainglorious assertions of the Knights of the Blended Rose."

Seven knights from each side appeared on the field and charged each other with blunted lances. When this failed to produce a single mock casualty, the lances were abandoned in favor of pistols, which the combatants fired into the air while riding furiously back and forth.

At the height of the battle, the field marshall rode in between the knights, assuring them that their ladies were abundantly satisfied that their honor had been successfully defended. Joining company, the two bands of knights paraded before the pavilions, saluting the ladies and General Howe.

Now, the whole assembly marched up a broad avenue overhung with flowered arches garishly decorated with scenes from ancient mythology. They ascended a long stairway to the front of the mansion, and when all of them had finally crowded into the hall, a set of doors was opened, revealing an immense, elaborately decorated ballroom. The orchestra struck up a minuet and the ladies danced, first with their knights, and then with their squires, before the rest of the company joined in.

At half-past ten o'clock the windows along one side of the room were suddenly thrown open and a dazzling display of fireworks shot up from the lawn below. As they subsided, another brilliant set of what appeared to be fireworks illuminated the distant horizon at the north end of Philadelphia. The sound of cannons filled the night air and the guests enthusiastically applauded such a clever arrangement of pyrotechnics. The latter display, however, turned out to be a company of American infantry headed by Captain Allan McLane who had set fire to the abatis connecting the northern line of the British defenses. Fire was exchanged, but the Americans escaped into the night, having ruined the evening for many of the British officers. The ladies, however, were entertained with the illusion that this had indeed been a part of the evening's entertainment.

The guests returned to the dance, but at midnight still another set of doors was opened at one end of the ballroom, and a vast dining hall was revealed. Two tables covered with an incredible assortment of food stretched the length of the room. In addition to fifty pyramids of jellies, syllabub, cakes, and sweetmeats, there were over 1,600 other dishes not including the great tureens of soups and stews. All of this was served by twenty-four black slaves dressed in silver collars and bracelets that derived from André's peculiar notion of Moorish costume.

By two o'clock the supper was coming to an end, but the party was far from over. After numerous toasts and a rousing chorus of "God Save the King," several of the company set to serious drinking while others drifted back to the ballroom to dance. At the first hint of dawn the guests began to disperse, though the sun was well up by the time Rebecca Franks, the Queen of the Burning Mountain, boarded her carriage for town.

If patriotic Americans were appalled by this show conducted while Washington's men starved at Valley Forge, there was an equal number of Loyalists who thought it a shameful excess. The participants in the revel, however, were quite proud of themselves; they had successfully carried off what even their critics agreed had been one of the grandest parties in history.

The British garrison had barely recovered when news came that Congress had concluded a treaty with France that would officially bring the French into the war on the American side. In London the decision was made to abandon Philadelphia in favor of stronger fortifications at New York. Howe returned to England in the afterglow of the Meschianza, and on June 18 Clinton and the British forces marched north out of the city. General Washington, however, quickly followed and, a few days later at Monmouth, New Jersey, the well-fed British were soundly defeated by an army that had barely survived the winter. Congress, the Continental army, and those Patriots who had fled in 1777, now flocked back into Philadelphia with a firm resolve never to let that city fall into British hands again. Loyalist high society, and a few Patriot belles, wistfully noted the passing of the British occupation.

The American general, Anthony Wayne, wrote to a friend on the twelfth of July:

> Tell those Philadelphia ladies who attended Howe's assemblies and levees, that the heavenly, sweet, pretty redcoats—the accomplished gentlemen of the guards and grenadiers, have been humbled on the plains of Monmouth. The knights of the Blended Roses, and of the Burning Mount—have resigned their laurels to rebel officers, who will lay them at the feet of *those* virtuous daughters of America who cheerfully gave up ease and affluence in a city, for liberty and peace of mind in a cottage.

But Wayne was either a romantic or badly misinformed. Among the affluent class of Philadelphia, few had fled the city, and none of those who remained—especially the attractive young ladies—had given up their ease. In exchange for hospitality, political differences were overlooked, and even patriotic Philadelphians were inclined to forget, for a while, that the pleasant and sociable British officers were the enemy. Events immediately following the American reoccupation of the city would also serve to demonstrate that Wayne had been engaging in a pleasant fiction.

As soon as the Americans returned and Philadelphia was reestablished as the capital, it was decided that a ball should be organized in honor of the treaty between the United States and France. Martha Washington was the official hostess of the affair. The question was immediately raised as to whether or not the ladies who had attended the Meschianza should be invited. Indignant Patriots denounced the Philadelphia belles for conspiring with the enemy, but as the guest list was being made out, it was widely agreed that a Philadelphia party without the likes of Rebecca Franks and Peggy Shippen would in fact be no party at all.

On the evening of the ball, the young ladies who had cavorted with the British officers a few short weeks before now greeted the Americans as old friends, hoping that the social life of the town would not falter in their presence. Rebecca dutifully paid her respects to Mrs. Washington and seemed less concerned that it was a patriotic affair than with the possibility that it might turn out to be a dull evening. Among the American officers were several admirers, but the elegant style of the British had turned her head. Bored by what she considered to be the excessive political concerns of the Patriots, Rebecca's contempt grew and revealed itself in a highly developed sense of mischief.

The principal event at this ball was the exchanging of the black and white cockades, or badges, which soldiers wore on their hats, signifying the joining of the French and American armies. After the ceremony when the party had returned to dancing, Rebecca bribed a servant to acquire the symbolic cockades and to fetch a dog from the neighborhood. Tying the knots around the dog's neck, she sent it running through the ballroom at the height of the party. The Washingtons were furious, but General Lafayette and the young American officers were inclined to instant forgiveness, especially since it was immediately suspected that the fair Rebecca Franks was the culprit.

If it seems a bit peculiar that Rebecca's behavior was tolerated at a time when tempers were running high, it must be remembered that she was not only a welcome figure at society functions, but was beautiful, well-bred, and an heiress in her own right, quite apart from the fortunes of her father. In short, she was to make a highly desirable wife for some prospective suitor. This was not lost on the young officers who, despite their own strong beliefs in the American cause, were hopeful that the conflict would soon be over and the time would come when political differences between Patriot and Loyalist would be forgotten. At such time Rebecca's British sympathies would matter very little.

Of course, Rebecca was equally aware of this situation, and even if she had no intention of becoming the wife of an American Patriot, she realized that there was some value in playing off the ardor of the men who surrounded her. Already a practiced coquette, Rebecca tempered her usual sarcasm with enough flirtation to keep everyone interested.

If those who courted Rebecca's favors were able to overlook her former associations and the vehemence with which she occasionally criticized the American cause, the harassed members of Congress were not similarly inclined. Protected as she was by her social connections, there was very little that could be done about her. Her father, on the other hand, was a different matter.

Now that the Americans were back in Philadelphia, Franks's subcontractors were demanding payment and accusing him of mishandling the financial affairs assigned to him by Congress. Wishing to avoid any blame for what was a quaint and unworkable agreement in the first place, Congress invented the convenient fiction that Franks must have been guilty of some indiscretion, though the facts plainly indicated that he was simply a man caught in the middle of a bad situation. With one eye on Rebecca's rather inimical behavior, Congress further reasoned that Franks must have been collaborating with the British, though, again, there was no evidence to support this.

With his own business rapidly failing, and in desperate need of the money owed him, Franks was forced to communicate secretly with the British. Absurd though it may seem, Congress was demanding that he collect these funds, but they refused to allow him to correspond directly with the British. Bills for payment sent legally through congressional channels died in indifference or mountains of red tape.

Finally the Americans intercepted a letter that Franks had written on October 18, 1778. In addition to its usual request for payment, it contained current market prices in Philadelphia, but absolutely no intelligence that might be of use to the enemy. Unfortunately near the end, he commented on the recent acquittal of a friend on charges of treason: "People are taken and confined at the pleasure of every scoundrel. Oh, in what a situation Britain has left its friends." This was sufficient for a Congress whose mind was already made up about Franks. He was stripped of his office, arrested, and thrown into jail. Let out on bail after a week, he was finally brought to trial in April 1779 on a misdemeanor charge of giving intelligence to the enemy. For lack of any substantiating evidence the jury quickly brought in a verdict of not guilty. But David Franks was only nominally a free man. Although he had been relieved of his responsibilities, he was still in the impossible position of owing Congress and his agents for 500,000 meals already consumed by British prisoners.

As usual, David's problems had little effect on his daughter. The very week he was sitting in jail, Rebecca appeared at a grand society ball, and her speech was no less guarded though her father was under suspicion of treason. Lieutenant Colonel Jack Steward of Maryland, who had known Rebecca since before the war, was the first to feel her sting. Hoping to impress the lady, he came sweeping into the ballroom dressed in a suit of scarlet. "I have adopted your colors, my Princess, the better to secure a courteous reception," he said. "Deign to smile on a true knight." Rebecca calmly turned her back to him and, in a loud voice, exclaimed to everyone in the room, "How the ass glories in the lion's skin." Steward was crestfallen, and though several Patriots stormed out of the room in anger, the party went on.

An account of Rebecca's sarcasm on this particular evening was immediately published in a local newspaper, which noted her as "a lady well-known in the Tory world." With her father out on bail pending trial, Rebecca might have done well to ignore the article, but in a succeeding issue of the paper there appeared the following reply:

There are many people so unhappy in their dispositions that, like the dog in the manger, they can neither enjoy the innocent pleasures of life themselves nor let others, without grumbling and growling, participate in them. Hence it is we frequently observe hints and anecdotes in your paper respecting the commanding officer, head-quarters, and Tory ladies. This mode of attacking characters is really admirable, and equally as polite as conveying slander and defamation by significant nods, winks, and shrugs. Poor beings indeed, who plainly indicate to what species of animals they belong, by the baseness of their conduct.

To defend her "innocent pleasures" at such a time, and in the public press, was of course callous and ill-advised, though it seemed to matter little to her that her own father was suffering under the burden of her peculiar fame.

Throughout the remainder of 1779 and 1780, Rebecca kept right on going to parties while her father pleaded with the British and Congress to secure payment for his debts. In October 1780 he was arrested again under an act "to apprehend suspected persons," though he was again released for lack of evidence. With harassment becoming a daily occurrence, Franks realized that he would never have peace until the British paid him, and he requested Congress to allow him to go to New York. He wrote that his daughter would like to accompany him and "would be very happy in taking a view of the Mall, or having a ramble under the holy old trees of Broadway." Congress responded by exiling both David Franks and his daughter permanently to New York, requiring that they post a £200,000 security that they would not "return again to any of these United States during the continuance of the present war." To David the exile was disheartening, but at least it finally presented him with a chance of getting his money. For Rebecca, exile afforded a pleasant change of scenery and reunion with her British admirers. Franks's property was not confiscated nor was he subjected to the usual persecution by the Philadelphia mobs, though he was forced to sell his considerable library and most of his furniture to make up the outrageous security demanded by Congress. His Jewish associates, who well understood his dilemma, became distant and silent lest they become somehow implicated in Franks's problems.

Rebecca had more than her ramble on Broadway. Taking up where she left off at the Meschianza two years earlier, she became once again the favorite of New York's British military society. In several letters to her sister Abigail, she commented on all the parties and excursions for which she was in constant demand. She was highly impressed by nobility and at one point noted that she was being courted by no less than three titled gentlemen simultaneously, "one with an income of £26,000 per year!"

Once upon returning to the city from the country estate of the Van Hornes on the Hudson, Rebecca wrote complaining about her father. She seemed ignorant of the fact that he was waging a private war with the British paymasters.

> You will think I have taken up my abode for the summer at Mrs. Van Horne's, but on the contrary, this day I return to the disagreeable, hot town, much against my will, and the inclination of the family. I cannot however bear papa's being so much alone, and he will not be persuaded to quit the city, though I am sure he can have no business to keep him there. Two nights he staid with us, which is all I have seen him since I left home. I am quite angry with him.

Her singular concern for her own comfort was held in abeyance on at least one occasion, however. She must have had some feeling for the members of her family, for upon hearing that her older brother Moses was about to join the British army she expressed her firm resolve on the matter to her sister:

> Was he ten or twelve years younger I should not have the smallest objection,—but 'tis too late for him to enter into such a life,—and after being commanded from post to pillar by every brat of a boy who may chance to be longer in the service. Tomorrow I shall write to him and make use of every argument I am mistress of to dissuade him from so mad a project, which I hope will arrive in time to prevent it, for if he once enters I would be the first to oppose his quitting it—as I ever lov'd a steady character. The danger of the war I have in measure reconciled myself to. 'Tis only his age I object to and the disagreeable idea of his being sent the Lord knows where. If he does enter, which I hope to God he may not, I wish he may join the 17th, or else get into the Dragoons—the latter I think he'll prefer on account of his lameness.

For the most part, though, Rebecca's letters concerned themselves with her favorite topics. She was less than enthusiastic about New York society. She found several aspects of life there to be quite provincial. For example, she was thoroughly annoyed that New Yorkers considered it improper and unsafe for her to step out unchaperoned by an older woman. "We Philadelphians," she wrote, "knowing no harm, fear'd none." As she wrote to Abigail, the gay life in New York's drawing rooms was plainly not up to her standards.

By the bye, few ladies here know how to entertain company in their own houses, unless they introduce the card-table. Except at the Van Hornes, who are remarkable for their good sense and ease, I don't know a woman or girl who can chat above half an hour, and that on the form of a cap, the color of a ribbon, or the set of a hoop, stay, or jupon. I will do our ladies—that is, the Philadelphians—the justice to say, that they have more cleverness in the turn of an eye, than those of New York have in their whole composition. With what ease have I seen a Chew, a Penn, an Oswald, an Allen, and a thousand others, entertain a large circle of both sexes, the conversation, without the aid of cards, never flagging, not seeming in the least strained or stupid. Here—or, more properly speaking, in New York—you enter the room with a formal, set curtsy, and after the how-dos, things are finished; all's a dead calm till the cards are introduced, when you see pleasure dancing in the eyes of all the matrons, and they seem to gain new life.

Neither was Rebecca impressed by the courting habits of young New Yorkers:

The maidens, if they have favorite swains, frequently decline playing, for the pleasure of making love; for to all appearance it is the ladies, not the gentlemen, who nowadays show a preference. It is here, I fancy, always leap-year. For my part, who am used to quite another style of behavior, I cannot help showing surprise—perhaps they call it ignorance—when I see a lady single out her pet, and lean almost into his arms, at an assembly or a play-house, (which I give my honor I have too often seen both with the married and single), or hear one confess a partiality for a man, whom, perhaps, she has not seen three times: "Well! I declare he is a delightful creature, and I could love him for my husband!" one exclaims, or, "I could marry such a gentleman!" Indeed scandal says that, in the cases of most who have been married, the first advances came from the lady's side, or she got a male friend to introduce the intended victim and pass her off. This is really the case, and with me ladies thus lose half their charms.

Knowing Rebecca's past history, her ideal of the amorous game was one in which the lady held the upper hand, remaining temptingly aloof, while the gentleman meekly pursued, lavishing every attention at his disposal and expecting little if anything in return. The slightly shocked tone of this letter probably refers to her disgust at these young ladies who relinquished their control over the game.

At the advanced age of twenty-one, however, it was clear that Rebecca was growing tired of the chase. On one occasion she told Abigail that she had been "writing in the parlor quite *en dishabille*," when three British officers entered. Quickly throwing on a dressing gown, she continued to write, leaving the officers to sit in embarrassed silence. "You may imagine what an indifferent I am," she went on, "to continue writing, with beaus in the room; but so it is! I am not what I was." A few months after this was written in late 1781, Rebecca was engaged to Sir Henry Johnson.

The two had met at the Meschianza. Though Johnson was fairly young, he was the very essence of a gentleman and soldier of the old school, and though Lord Cornwallis once referred to him as "a wrong-headed blockhead," he was quiet, genteel, and an immensely wealthy member of the British aristocracy. In short, he had all the qualifications that Rebecca had been looking for in a husband. For his part, Sir Henry seems to have been one of those retiring men who live vicariously by surrounding themselves with aggressive and witty comrades. He could have found no more perfect wife than Rebecca Franks.

With the fall of Yorktown in late 1781, New York became one of the last remaining centers of British occupation. They would not evacuate the city until after the Treaty of Paris in 1783, though it was fairly clear by this point that the war was effectively over. British and American interest in the conflict immediately began to flag.

Not the least of those whose concern was on the wane were Sir Henry and Rebecca—if, in fact, either of them had ever given more than a moment's reflection to the issues or implications of the war. Sir Henry's thoughts turned to his native land, while Rebecca contemplated her future as the wife of an English lord—a life she had never experienced, but one to which she was thoroughly convinced she belonged. In January 1782 they were married in New York, and in the spring they sailed for Bath, England, and the Johnson estate.

After peace had been formally declared, David Franks was permitted to return to Philadelphia. No charges were brought against him, and for the most part, Congress was all too willing to forget the man whom they had treated so unjustly. Of course, Franks never obtained a fraction of the money that the British owed him, and in attempting to repay his provisioning agents, he was ruined financially, once and for all. Despite this, it is said that David remained genial and uncomplaining throughout his later years. Although it was partially Rebecca's fault that he ended up in such disfavor during the war, he never mentioned the fact and continued to speak in only the most glowing terms about his beloved daughter. Though both Abigail and, to a greater extent, Rebecca easily could have afforded to maintain their father after his bankruptcy, they simply ignored his difficulties. But as usual, David Franks never criticized. Fortunately he was accepted back into the Jewish elite in Philadelphia, and through small loans obtained from Michael Gratz, one of his fellow Sephardim, he managed to survive. He never saw Rebecca again, though it is said that they wrote to each other often.

Though the remainder and greater portion of her life was spent in England, Rebecca Franks remains an intriguing figure in American history and a notable example of the conflict between personal interests and social and political movements that so characterized the Revolutionary period. If Rebecca was self-centered like many people, her primary interest was in a way of life, not in what others might have seen as millennial issues. As one who stood so firmly for her own beliefs, shallow though many might consider them, her story and that of her father serve to remind that justice is rarely done by forcing the apolitical person into one or another ideological camp.

Ultimately, and as General Scott's anecdote seems to indicate, Rebecca would form a set of political opinions based on the experiences and considerations of a lifetime, but they would be as mixed as those which characterized her native city of Philadelphia during the war. Pride in the fantastic accomplishments of her former countrymen and unyielding loyalty to her love of British culture blended to produce this curious woman who could exclaim at one moment, "Would to God I too had been a Patriot," while at the same time she sat at the head of a family line that would one day stud the pages of *Burke's Peerage* and the records of the officer corps of the British Army.

10

Fritschen von Riedesel

IN THE MID-EIGHTEENTH CENTURY, much of Germany was divided into a jumbled patchwork of nearly 300 sovereign states, electorates, duchies, bishoprics, and dominions of various petty nobles. Additionally, there were over 1,400 estates of Imperial Knights holding many of the rights of sovereignty. Only nominally under the control of the Austrian and Prussian crowns, each of these principalities was governed by an autonomous local lord. A few were enlightened enough to consider the welfare of their subjects, though most were autocratic despots who lived extravagantly in imitation of the French court.

Because most of their subjects were either craftsmen or small farmers, and because the population of any one dominion was relatively small, there was a decided limit to the amount of wealth that the nobles could extract through taxation. As their profligacy grew in the late seventeenth and early eighteenth centuries, they turned more and more to the one resource left after everything else of value had been exhausted. They became businessmen specializing in the sale of men.

In short, this landed nobility provided mercenary armies for a price, and they were not particular as to how men were obtained or who the customers were. Volunteers made up the smallest portion, and most of these were professional adventurers. The rest were "pressed" into service in one way or another, either through bribery, tricks, or outright force. Most of the German princes unscrupulously provided armies at one time or another to any nation and even factions within nations who would pay the going price, often with horrible results. During the Seven Years' War, Hessian troops fought for both the British and the French; brothers and sons and fathers found themselves firing at each other across the field of battle.

The greatest number of mercenary troops who fought in America was provided by the dukedom of Hesse-Cassel and the county of Hesse-Hanau; thus, the word Hessian came to denote all the German mercenaries in America. This misnomer greatly disturbed the soldiers and commanders of the other four principalities, however, for they saw themselves as citizens of independent states. The duke of Anhalt-Zerbst, for example, would refer to the subjects in neighboring Hesse-Cassel as "foreigners." The first of these independent states to conclude a treaty with England to send troops to America was the dukedom of Brunswick-Luneburg.

This first German contingent, called the Brunswickers, left Wolfenbuttel on the morning of February 22, 1776 and traveled over land and sea to Portsmouth, England, for embarkation to America. At their head was the thirty-eight-year-old Colonel Baron Friedrich Adolphus von Riedesel, a professional soldier with twenty-four years of service to the dukes of Hesse-Cassel and Brunswick. This first army departed with 2,282 men, 77 wives, and an uncounted number of children walking behind the baggage wagons. More than a year later the wife of the Baron von Riedesel and her children would follow, too.

The Baroness Frederika Charlotte Luise von Riedesel was the strikingly beautiful second daughter of Commissary General von Massow, a senior officer in service to Duke Ferdinand of Brunswick. Her marriage to the baron had been arranged in 1763, though the two had known each other for some years before this and were very much in love. "Fritschen," as her family called her, was not of noble birth, but her family was wealthy enough to raise her with all the advantages of nobility, including a thorough training in literary skills that, one day, would aid her in leaving behind a remarkable record of her experiences in America.

Fritschen had not left with her husband because she was pregnant at the time, and while the baron was still in England, he was informed that she had given birth to another girl. One month after the baron's ship left Portsmouth, Madame von Riedesel was on the road bound for Calais with her two older daughters, Augusta and Frederika, and the infant Caroline at her breast.

Throughout the fall of 1776 the baroness attempted to find a berth for her family on board a ship headed for Quebec. After many disappointments, she finally located one reported to be leaving from

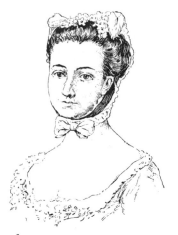

Fritschen von Riedesel
Courtesy, Historical Pictures Service, Chicago

London, but she arrived to find that it had already sailed. With winter fast approaching, the Atlantic crossing would become impossible, so the baroness and her children settled in London to await the spring.

Fritschen spoke only French and German, and though she was entertained by London aristocracy and was even received by the king and queen, she was mistreated by shopkeepers and street crowds who ridiculed her for her inability to communicate in English. Also, as a German aristocrat, she dressed in emulation of the ladies of the French court and, in particular, Marie Antoinette. To say the least, the French were not popular in England, and, on one occasion, she was surrounded by a crowd of English sailors who pointed at her dress yelling, "French whore!" Needless to say, Fritschen soon had dresses made in the English fashion and studied the language with a vengeance. By the time she left England, she could read the newspapers and carry on all necessary business in English.

Finally, in April 1777, the baroness secured passage aboard the man-of-war, *Blonde,* which set sail from Portsmouth, and after eight weeks at sea, the ship dropped anchor at Quebec. When the other ships in the harbor heard of the baroness's arrival, they fired cannon salutes in her honor. The baron had been promoted to general, and now Fritschen was "frau general"; toward noon of July 11 a British boat, manned by twelve sailors dressed in white and wearing silver helmets and green sashes, came to transport her to land. They carried a letter from her husband, informing her that he had departed Quebec to join his army farther south, and implying that she should await his return. Fritschen had come too far to wait any longer and determined to set out immediately to meet her "Fritz."

Before the Revolutionary War took place, there was little information about America in Germany. Editors would occasionally invent outrageous fictions about the new world as filler for their newspapers—secure in the knowledge that few could contradict them—though accurate accounts were lacking as was any genuine interest. Fritschen had read a few of the travelers' accounts written or translated into German or French, but many of these presented exaggerated pictures of either a paradise or a bleak wilderness crawling with savages. Common folk wisdom among her friends back in Brunswick had it that the continent was a vast, dismal swamp, the Indians were cannibals—especially fond of children— and that the English in America dined regularly on insects and lizards or, at best, cats and dogs. Later the baroness would confess that she had believed a certain amount of this. As she approached Quebec, she tried to submerge her fears in the anticipation she felt for her husband.

General von Riedesel and his Brunswickers now formed one of the principal units of the army under the command of General "Gentleman Johnny" Burgoyne. After four days of hard traveling, the baroness finally found her husband's unit near the town of Chambly, and though the reunion was as poignant and satisfying as Fritschen had hoped, her husband had to return to his army. Within two days, she was sent back to the town of Three Rivers, feeling, as she said, "alone and deserted with [my] children, in a foreign land among strangers."

Three Rivers, located on the St. Lawrence River about halfway between Quebec and Montreal, was a charming town that had preserved much of the flavor of Old France. Madame von Riedesel noted the beautiful view of the river which it commanded as well as the clean, whitewashed houses and the flourishing agriculture and animal husbandry of the area.

Much of Fritschen's time there was spent in caring for her children and battling with British paymasters. The von Riedesels were committed to subsisting on the allotments promised under the British treaty with Brunswick rather than dipping into their family estates, though local paymasters, unsure of their positions, often proved miserly. Of course, the baroness was no less unsure of her present situation, though she was not to be intimidated either by obstinate clerks or the terrors of the battlefield. Fritschen was fiercely determined that her family would survive this experience and return to Germany, preferably victorious, though at least with high spirits, good health, and considerable additions to the family coffers. She was well aware of her own physical fortitude and intelligence and was not above using her obvious beauty and charm to protect her interests. A British paymaster was simply no match for her. If there were fears and misgivings about this whole enterprise, as there often were, there was never despair. Fritschen was too strong-willed and fond of life to succumb to this.

Having received the money owed her by the British, Fritschen begged her husband to let her join him. He finally acquiesced, and on August 14, 1777 the baroness and her children arrived at Fort Edward on the Hudson River, south of Lake George. It had taken less than two weeks for the baroness to travel the distance from Three Rivers to the fort. By the time she arrived, Burgoyne had placed the baron in charge of an expedition that was to travel south to capture supplies at Bennington, Vermont.

General von Riedesel did not join the battle himself but sent two Hessian colonels in command of over 1,000 men. Directing the strategy and supply trains from Fort Miller, von Riedesel had his plans constantly interfered with by Burgoyne, who made disastrous changes in the army's route. Eight miles from Bennington they were met by 700 Americans. Sporadic fighting occurred for the next two days, and though more German reinforcements arrived, by the afternoon of August 16 the surviving British and German troops were routed and forced to flee back to Fort Miller. Of the 200 Brunswick dragoons sent to Bennington, only twenty-nine returned.

On the eighteenth General von Riedesel rejoined his wife at Fort Edward, greatly saddened by the failure of this expedition and furious over Burgoyne's interference. Nevertheless, Fritschen wrote:

> We passed very happily the [next] three weeks together. The country around us was beautiful. . . . We had for our lodgings a dwelling called the Red House. When the weather was fine, we dined under the trees, and if not, in a barn, where planks were laid upon some

casks, to serve as a table. Here I tasted, for the first time, bear's flesh, and found it delightful. We often were in want of everything, and I was nevertheless very happy and content, for I was with my children, and was sure of the attachment of those who surrounded me.

In regard to the disaster at Bennington, however, she merely reports it as an "unfortunate engagement" because of which her husband was able to rejoin her at Fort Edward.

Now Burgoyne planned to march south to take Albany, and, at first, the baron was elated that a major step in the campaign was about to be taken. By the end of August, however, the Americans under Benedict Arnold had taken Fort Stanwix. There had been a mass defection of the Indians from the British, and it turned out that there were few Loyalists in the area who were willing to flock to the British side. His optimism fading about the march to Albany, the baron proposed to send Madame von Riedesel and the children back to Canada. But Fritschen was stubborn, and after several appeals the baron permitted her to stay. On September 11 the army broke camp and the baroness wrote, "In the beginning, all went well, we thought that there was little doubt of our being successful, and of reaching 'the promised land,' [Albany] and when on the passage across the Hudson, general Burgoyne exclaimed, 'Britons never retrograde,' our spirits rose mightily."

The baroness's aristocratic spirits, however, were somewhat depressed by at least two circumstances of the British camp. Burgoyne traveled with his mistress who was the wife of one of his commissaries. This placed Fritschen in an awkward position because when she invited the general to dine, it was expected that his lady be invited also. There is no record of the commissary's opinion of all this, but the baroness had to suffer the embarrassment of a situation that was completely contrary to her notions of proper behavior. Fritschen was from a military family and therefore, not naive about the ways of men in war. Nevertheless, when confronted with actual examples of this unchivalrous behavior she would become greatly incensed; there were, after all, correct forms to observe.

Even more shocking:

I observed with surprise, that the wives of the officers were beforehand informed of all the military plans; and I was so much the more struck with it, as I remembered with how much secrecy all dispositions were made in the armies of Duke Ferdinand, during the seven-years' war. Thus the Americans anticipated all our movements, and expected us wherever we arrived: and this of course injured our affairs.

It was very disconcerting that the Americans maintained absolute secrecy, though apparently the effects of this difference never seem to have made an impression on Burgoyne. The baroness was too familiar with traditional German discipline on this point not to be appalled.

Skirmishes along the road were frequent, though minor, and usually ended to the advantage of the British. By September 19, the royal forces were entrenched at a place called Freeman's Farm near Saratoga. A small log cabin with a fireplace was hurriedly built for Fritschen and the children a few miles from the encampment. The baron stayed with his troops, though he dined with his family each evening. Every morning the baroness would don her riding habit—shocking to everyone else, for the costume included trousers—and travel to the camp where she would have breakfast with her husband. On the morning of October 7, however, she noticed more activity than usual in the camp, and on the way back to her house she saw obvious preparations for an encounter. Generals Burgoyne, Fraser, and Phillips were to dine with her that afternoon, but at the appointed hour General Fraser was carried in on a litter, mortally wounded in the stomach. The Americans were steadily advancing on the British positions.

> The table, which was already prepared for dinner, was immediately removed, and a bed placed in its stead for the general. I sat terrified and trembling in a corner. The noise grew more alarming, and I was in continual agony and tremour, while thinking that my husband might soon also be brought in, wounded like general Fraser.

The baron returned later that evening and allayed her fears, though she noted that "We poor females had been told that our troops had been victorious; but I well saw, by the melancholy countenance of my husband, that it was quite the contrary." Before returning to camp that night the baron confirmed her doubts, and Fritschen set to packing up their baggage.

Under cover of darkness, the British retreated from Freeman's Farm and reached Saratoga by early the next evening. Burgoyne stopped the army constantly, drawing up his lines, counting his artillery, and engaging in a number of useless formalities. At one point, he permitted a troop of 200 American reconnaissance scouts to escape. Burgoyne was a master of indecision and the baron's frustrations grew as his own recommendations were ignored and their peril increased. Rain was falling in torrents throughout the journey, movement of the artillery pieces was extremely slow, and General von Riedesel hadn't slept in two days.

Fritschen observed that in the confusion of this retreat, Burgoyne seemed to have lost his head. What should have been an orderly withdrawal turned into a disorganized rout. The baron offered to protect the army's rear, if only haste would be made, but Burgoyne procrastinated, spent his nights in drinking bouts with his mistress and ignored the advice of his senior officers. Worst of all, Burgoyne had not followed up his orders for the distribution of rations, and by the time the troops reached Saratoga they were starving. It seems that the baroness had been feeding several of the officers out of her own provisions, but now that these were gone she called Burgoyne's adjutant general aside and demanded that he bring this to the general's attention. "In less than a quarter of an hour," Fritschen reported,

> General Burgoyne came towards me, thanked me most pathetically, for having reminded him of his duty. He added that a general whose orders were not obeyed, was much to be pitied. I replied, that I begged his pardon, for having meddled in the affairs with which a woman had nothing to do; but that I could not forebear saying what I had expressed, when I saw so many gallant officers in need of everything, while I was destitute of the means of assisting them. He thanked me again, (though I really believe he has never forgiven me).

On October 9 the battle at Saratoga began in earnest, and the baroness and her children retired to a small house on the north side of the town. Several other families joined them along with a number of wounded soldiers. Seeing all this activity around the house, the Americans thought that it must be the headquarters; and an artillery barrage was laid in that lasted for three days. Fritschen huddled in the cellar with the others, including many dead and dying, while the cannonballs systematically destroyed the house above. Panicked troops constantly tried to take shelter with them, but, fearful for her children, the baroness would throw herself across the entrance. Neither a British nor a German soldier would knock aside a baroness. There was almost no food and only a little wine to drink, and since the intense fire confined them to the cellar, it was fouled with excrement and the stench of the dead. One brave soldier's wife stole out to get water from the river, whereupon the Americans on the other side held their fire. Fritschen would note the gentlemanly conduct of the Americans in this matter, but when the baron suggested that she be sent to the American camp to keep her and the children from danger, she declared that "nothing would be more painful to me, than to live on good terms with those whom [the baron] was fighting; upon which he consented that I should continue to follow the army."

During these three days Fritschen received brief visits from her husband and spent most of the time caring for the growing number of wounded, stretching the meager rations to feed them, and comforting her children. By October 11, the British position had become untenable; losses were heavy, supplies were running low, and Burgoyne ordered a retreat. The baroness remained in her cellar, while it took the army almost four more days to retreat eight miles to a little plateau northwest of Saratoga. But the Americans held all the escape routes, and by the thirteenth it was commonly agreed among the British and German generals that further retreat was now impossible. For two days capitulation proposals were exchanged between Burgoyne and Gates, and on the morning of the seventeenth, Burgoyne surrendered his armies to the Americans. Under the agreement the officers were to be exchanged for captured American officers as soon as possible, the troops were to be returned to Europe, and terms such as capitulation and prisoner-of-war were not to be used. Rather this was a convention, and Burgoyne's armies were to be known as the Troops of the Convention. The baron's groom arrived shortly thereafter to invite Fritschen and the children to join him. Seated in the calash, they rode off toward the American camp.

The baroness seems to have experienced less concern for their defeat than joy that the crises and anxieties of the past few months were over. Her family was still safe and together, and that was of the utmost importance. Any apprehension she may have had over this turn of events was immediately lessened, as she related:

> While riding through the American camp, I was gratified to observe that no body looked at us with disrespect, but, on the contrary, greeted us, and seemed touched at the sight of a captive mother with three children. I must candidly confess that I did not present myself,

though so situated, with much courage to the enemy, for the thing was entirely new to me.

Upon arriving in the camp, she was invited to the tent of General Gates, whom she found in pleasant conversation with Burgoyne. Burgoyne proclaimed that she could now "be quiet and free from all apprehension of danger," and the baroness replied that, "I should indeed be reprehensible, if I felt any anxiety, when our general felt none, and was on such friendly terms with General Gates." That evening she was the guest of General Schuyler who "regaled" her, as she said, "with smoked tongues, which were excellent, with beefsteaks, potatoes, fresh butter, and bread. Never did a dinner give me so much pleasure as this."

Schuyler invited the von Riedesels to visit his family at their house in Albany, and they spent three days there with Burgoyne. Fritschen noted that they did not enter that city with a victorious army, as they had hoped:

> The reception, however, which we met with from general Schuyler, his wife, and daughters, was not like the reception of enemies, but of the most intimate friends. They loaded us with kindness; and they behaved in the same manner toward general Burgoyne, though he had ordered their splendid establishment to be burnt, and without any necessity, as it was said.

Among such enemies, Fritschen could begin to feel somewhat more secure about the future.

For the next several days the von Riedesels traveled overland, following the German troops to Cambridge, Massachusetts, supposedly to await transport to Europe. The baron brooded continually over the defeat and the possibility that he would receive some of the blame for Burgoyne's mishandling of the campaign. By now his health was much impaired from exposure and exhaustion and, in fact, he would not fully recover for several years. Along the route he was greatly annoyed by curious Americans who constantly besieged their calash to get a look at the German general and his family. Fritschen would leap out to satisfy the crowds and to keep them from tearing the cloth covering of the wagon which, as she noted, "looked more like a cart in which wild animals are conveyed." "But I must say, in justice," she wrote, "that the Americans were civil, and seemed much pleased that I spoke their language."

A few days later the baron was ill, and the American sentinels outside their door were drunk and noisy. They ignored the baron's pleas for quiet, but when Madame von Riedesel made the same request there was immediate silence, "which proves," she said, "that the Americans also respect our sex." These first impressions were not inaccurate, nor would Fritschen retract her basic feeling of good will toward Americans, though there would be several unpleasant experiences in the years to come.

Since winter was already setting in, it was decided that the convention troops would remain in Cambridge until spring when the Atlantic crossing would be safe.

The von Riedesels managed to secure an old farmhouse in that city—which the baroness loved—and life settled into a comfortable pattern. Fritschen visited about the town making friends with other Loyalists, entertained nightly, and even threw a ball for her husband's birthday at which there were eighty guests, and "God Save the King" was sung with enthusiasm.

About Boston she said, "It is quite a fine city, but the inhabitants are outrageously patriotic." General Schuyler's son-in-law taunted her, saying that General von Riedesel's head should be cut off, pickled, and sent to the next British raiding party that burned an American village. She also related a story concerning a Bostonian "Republican" who threatened to kill his brother because he was a Loyalist. Such examples of outrageous patriotism must have been typical of the baroness's experiences in her forays into Boston, and it is likely that she kept to her house in Cambridge. Since she was surrounded by German and British friends, it seems to have been an agreeable time for her.

As spring approached and plans for the embarkation were being made, Burgoyne and von Riedesel discovered that the Americans intended to violate the terms of the convention. Though Burgoyne had promised that the same units would never fight in America again, Congress was sure that the men would simply be formed into new regiments in England and immediately returned to the war. To add to the baron's consternation, he received a letter from Duke Ferdinand of Brunswick stating that the German troops should either be kept in America or exiled to the Isle of Wight. If they returned to Germany, they might discourage enlistments in future mercenary armies. Whatever their official designation, the convention troops were now prisoners of war. Most of the Brunswickers would remain in American prison camps until 1783. All but abandoned by his own sovereign, von Riedesel had no choice but to remain behind with his troops. It would be three more years before he would be exchanged, and he would never see action against the Americans again.

By the summer of 1778, the imprisoned army and its officers had worn thin their welcome in Cambridge. Food and supplies were growing short and the New Englanders saw no reason why they should deny themselves to provide for the captive enemy. General Clinton, commander of the British forces in New York, was supposed to pay for the support of his imprisoned comrades-in-arms, but when he finally refused, Congress decided that the convention troops should be moved to a more rural location where they could provide for themselves. In November the order was sent that they were to be relocated to Virginia.

The journey to Charlottesville took more than two months, owing to the rain and snow of an early winter and the slow progress of the now tattered and bedraggled German regiments. The baron had purchased an "elegant English coach" for Fritschen's and the children's comfort, but it was top heavy and in constant danger of tipping over on the rough roads. They traveled at a steady pace, stopping for a one-day rest only once every four days. These stops were the only times when there was enough food, for though they had adequate provisions in their baggage train, it often lagged behind them by as much as a full day.

Shortly after their departure from Cambridge, they came to Hartford, Connecticut, where, the baroness was horrified to learn, her husband had invited Lafayette to dine with them. Their baggage was still far back on the road and, knowing the French general to be a great gourmet, Fritschen was perplexed as to how to make a fine show out of the meager provisions she had with her. Apparently she found a way, however, for she noted that the dinner did indeed answer Lafayette's expectations. They rapidly became friends, spending the evening speaking in French.

A few days later, Fritschen stopped at what she called "a pretty little town," probably in the Berkshire Mountains, where they were quartered in the house of a woman who sold fresh meat. As usual the provisions wagon was far behind, and the children were hungry. "Let me have some, I will pay you liberally," Fritschen begged the woman. But the woman snapped her fingers in the baroness's face, "You shall not have a morsel of it. Why have you left your country to slay us and rob us of our property? Now that you are our prisoners, it is our turn to vex you." The baroness made no reply, but her youngest daughter pulled at the woman's skirts and pleaded that she and her sisters were very hungry. The woman's heart melted a bit and she gave the girls some eggs, but she remained adamant with the baroness. In the presence of so much food, however, Fritschen was not to be bested. Quietly she retired to a corner of the kitchen fireplace where

> I made tea, and the hostess looked at our teapot with a longing eye, for the Americans were very fond of that beverage; yet they had stoutly resolved not to drink any more, the tax on tea, as is well known, having been the immediate cause of the contest with Great Britain. I offered her, however, a cup, and presented her with a paper case full of tea.

Fritschen had found the key, for the woman immediately brought up enough food from the cellar for a large meal and gave the von Riedesels "three neat rooms, with very good beds" for the night.

The von Riedesels next lodged with a boatman's family whose wife Fritschen termed a "real termagant, and anti-Loyalist," and "a shrew." It seems that the woman threw the von Riedesels out of her house in the midst of a violent storm, and they were forced to cross the Hudson in a small boat which nearly capsized several times. On the opposite shore they received no better treatment. At first a Colonel Osborn ejected two of the general's aides-de-camp from his fireside saying, "Is it not enough that I give you shelter, ye wretched Loyalists?" Fritschen described him as "surly," and coarsely dressed with a scraggly beard. On the following day, Fritschen was invited to take coffee with the colonel and his wife, but as she rose to leave the colonel asked, "Are you afraid of me?" "No, sir," replied Fritschen,

> "I fear nobody, not even a figure as ugly as you were yesterday." Instead of waxing wroth, he softened; and taking me by the hand, he begged me to sit down again, next to his wife. "I am not so rude as you imagine," said he, "I like you, and if I were not married, I cannot tell but I might fall in love with you."—"Do you believe that I would encourage your affection?"—"As for that we should see: I am very rich; this whole estate is mine; my wife, you see, is old: you will do well, therefore, to remain here."

Throughout the following week the von Riedesels enjoyed the colonel's excellent hospitality, but Fritschen remained uncertain as to whether that was a proposal of marriage or something else.

The baroness's account of the journey was spare. Overwhelmed by the strangeness and exertions of the 700-mile trek through Massachusetts, Connecticut, New York, New Jersey, Pennsylvania, Maryland, and Virginia, she simply noted, "We passed through a picturesque country, but of so wild a character, that it left awful impressions. The traveling was dangerous, the roads being almost impassable; and we suffered not only from the cold, but from want." In the middle of February 1779 the baroness arrived at her destination, an estate called Colle near Charlottesville, Virginia, where the baron had arrived with his troops some three weeks before. The von Riedesels had previously arranged to lease Colle from its owner, an Italian physician named Signor Philip Mazzei who was about to depart for Europe to assume his post as financial agent for the state of Virginia.

Across a narrow valley, on a slightly higher hill than the one on which Colle was situated, rose the white columns of Thomas Jefferson's beloved Monticello. Mazzei's and Jefferson's orchards were in full bloom when the baroness arrived, and the green mist of sprouting forests spread across the hills of this beautiful part of Virginia. Their house, though small, appeared adequate. Mazzei and his shrewish wife and daughter were still in residence, however, and now the Mazzeis and the von Riedesels and their twenty servants and aides crowded into the small building. The co-existence was an unpleasant experience for the von Riedesels. On the verge of divorce, the Mazzeis fought constantly and their daughter was so spoiled as to be unbearable. Fritschen was overjoyed when the family soon departed for Paris.

In early March the warm spring weather suddenly turned back to winter, and frosts killed off the blooming orchards. Heavy winds and snowstorms came sweeping across the hills and nearly blew the "mansion house" of Colle apart. The baron set to work building a new house, probably with the help of Jefferson's architectural expertise, and by the end of April the family was comfortably installed in their new home.

On April 29 Jefferson noted in his personal records, "sold my pianoforte to General Riedesel who is to give me £100." Fritschen was an excellent musician, but it had been a long time since she had played the piano. The gift pleased her immensely as it did everyone else at Colle, for now there were "musical displays" in the evenings at which Fritschen would play along with other musicians in the German camp. Light songs and folk tunes were popular among the soldiers, but the baroness would command her audience by playing and singing arias from the operas.

But the German prisoners were not the only ones charmed by the baroness's musical abilities. Sometime in April the British Major General Phillips, who had been captured at Saratoga, held a dinner to which the von Riedesels and the Jeffersons were invited. Martha Jefferson was as charming and witty in her own way as was Fritschen, and she was also a fine musician, both on the piano and harpsichord. With so much in common the two women became instant friends. Though the baroness makes no mention of it in her journal, the Jeffersons and the von Riedesels spent many musical evenings together at Colle and Monticello.

The friendship was short-lived, however. In June Jefferson was elected governor of Virginia, and when he and his family left Charlottesville, Baron von Riedesel wrote them a regretful letter. Jefferson replied noting the "loss of the agreeable society . . . of which Madame Riedesel and yourself were an important part," and of Mrs. Jefferson's "regret on her separation from madame de Riedesel."

In fact, Thomas Jefferson must have been very fond of the von Riedesels, for shortly after taking the post of governor he did them a considerable favor. Fritschen and the children had enjoyed excellent health since their arrival in Virginia; in fact, the baroness was referred to as *embonpoint* meaning, simply, rather sexily voluptuous. But the general's health had improved little; he suffered frequently from dizziness and headaches. The doctors recommended the fashionable cure of "taking the waters" and suggested that he spend some time at Frederick-Spring, now called Berkeley Springs. The conditions of their confinement required the von Riedesels to stay in the area of Charlottesville, but Jefferson provided them with a formal letter of parole permitting them to travel anywhere in Virginia they pleased.

Frederick-Spring was not yet a resort, but simply a fairly wild place in the hills where the Virginian aristocracy set up elegant little camps while they took their cures, drinking and bathing in the mineral springs that abounded in the area. Fritschen thought that the waters actually did her husband very little good and feared that "he increased his disorder by washing his head." The baron remained ill and irritable and apparently kept to his tent most of the time. Fritschen, however, was more sociable, and in her morning forays to the springs she met several of those camping nearby. She mentioned that she became acquainted with "General Washington's family"—probably Martha and her granddaughters—and Mary Carroll, the wife of Charles Carroll of Carrollton whom she described as "a very amiable woman, and notwithstanding her great attachment to her country, we became great friends."

While at the springs, word came that General Phillips and von Riedesel were finally to be exchanged. Neither of them was optimistic about the possibility, but the baron returned to Charlottesville to dispose of all his household effects, and Fritschen left directly for York, Pennsylvania, where she was to meet her husband. At the invitation of Mary Carroll, she stopped at the estate of Mary's father-in-law, Doughoregan, near Annapolis: "After having passed a neat village, inhabited by Negroes, each of whom had a little garden near his hut, and knew some handicraft, we rode through a fine avenue towards the beautiful mansion-house, where the whole family waited for us and received us with great cordiality."

The Carroll family became very much enamoured of Fritschen, and she of them—all of them, that is, except for Charles, the first signer of the Declaration of Independence. Of him she wrote, "he was not very lovable, but rather brusque and miserly and not at all suited to his wife, who did not appear very happy." Nevertheless, when the baroness left Doughoregan over a week later, Mary made sure that she was loaded down with provisions.

> She furnished us with many things, which there was little prospect we should want for a long time; and that liberality was in reality superfluous, for the royalists received us with frank hospitality, from political sympathy, and those of opposite principles gave us a friendly welcome, merely from habit, for, in that country, it would be considered a crime to behave otherwise towards strangers.

The baroness finally rejoined her husband at York, and together with General Phillips they traveled on toward New York. Stopping at Elizabeth, New Jersey, across from Staten Island, the von Riedesels were in high spirits, so close to British New York and their impending exchange. During dinner, however, an officer commissioned by General Washington entered with a letter informing them that the exchange had been canceled, and that they must return to Virginia.

> The general [Phillips] gave way to the natural irritability of his

temper. Transported by passion, he started, and stamped and uttered the most injurious expressions against the members of congress. I was at first so terrified, that I could not say a word. The general came to me, and taking me by the hand, he said, "Do not lose courage, my dear madam; pray, follow my example: see how composed I am!" "Everyone," returned I, "manages his sorrows in his own way. I conceal mine in the recesses of my heart."

Phillips apologized and calmed down, but no one there, including Fritschen, could conceal his sadness.

After scarcely more than a day's rest, the baroness set off for Virginia. On the road to Bethlehem, Pennsylvania, she lodged one night with a family she had stayed with on the way north. They had impressed her as the most loyal subjects of the king, and she was anxious to be with them again. Now, however, she arrived to find the nephew of General Washington and several other American officers staying there, who

within three days, had brought about such a change in the opinions of our host, that not only were his daughters extremely affable towards the republican officers, but indulged them with the song of "God save great Washington; God damn the King." I could scarcely conceal my indignation, when I took leave of them the next morning.

Upon reaching Bethlehem, von Riedesel and Phillips received word that they could remain there until the problems of the exchange could be worked out. It seems that obstacles had arisen because the baron had left behind several debts in Charlottesville, and Phillips had left behind a number of insults. It took six weeks for enough money to be found and apologies to be made before Congress permitted them to return to Elizabeth. On the way, as ill-luck would have it, Fritschen's carriage broke down near the door of the family of "pretended" Loyalists. "I did not, however, spend the night under their roof," she protested, "and when they begged us to recommend them, and indulged in self-applause for their devotion to the king . . . I replied coldly, that I thought they did not want our recommendation; an answer that had more than one meaning."

Still von Riedesel and Phillips were not exchanged, though they were finally permitted to move into New York on parole. They arrived late one evening and were greeted by a soldier who led them to their supposedly "humble" quarters which actually turned out to be the Walton house, probably the most elegant house in the city at the time. It had been provided anonymously by General Tryon, royal governor of New York, because he was afraid that the baroness would not accept the favor otherwise. Lavish meals appeared regularly, and when Generals Clinton and Cornwallis came to call, they were entertained royally. Fritschen could not bear the thought of how much this was costing them and she demanded an accounting. It was then she was informed of Tryon's kindness.

Later the family was moved to a permanent residence which had been arranged for them by General Pattison, the British commandant of the city. It was a large three-story house just off the battery, one block from the fort where the baron spent much of his time. The house was elegantly done in mahogany with gorgeous furnishings confiscated from the Patriots and carpeting on the floors—something still considered an ostentatious luxury in Germany.

As the baroness reported, "I continued to be treated with excessive kindness, during the whole time I remained at New York, and I spent the winter very agreeably." She made many friends and apparently captured the hearts of the officers of the garrison, for in late January when the queen's birthday was to be celebrated, Fritschen was chosen to stand in for Queen Charlotte at the balls and festivities that were common on this holiday.

The title of "Queen of the Ball" was quite an honor, but it seems that Fritschen did not have first claim to it. The wife of General Cornwallis's adjutant was of noble birth and outranked the baroness. She was less popular than Fritschen, however. Because she was far advanced in pregnancy, the officers made the excuse that the round of balls would be too grueling for the poor lady, and so Fritschen was nominated instead.

The baroness herself was in somewhat of a "delicate condition," though not so far advanced as the British lady. In early March she met a Hessian general who had been a close friend when they were both very young. "Ha! ha!" he exclaimed, "what have you done with your elegant figure, your brilliant complexion, and your pretty tapered white hands? They are gone. . . . " No doubt they were, not because Fritschen had lost her beauty, but because by now she was large with child. She took the chiding good-naturedly, however, and begged the general "to take from me the advice, never to remind a lady of her past beauty, lest he should meet with many, who would not hear such things with as much indifference as myself."

On March 7, 1780 the baroness gave birth to her child—another girl. The prayed-for boy was to have been named Americus. "My husband wished very much for a son," Fritschen wrote, "but the baby was so pretty that we were soon consoled." They named her Amerika, and from then on she came to be referred to as Miss America. She was baptized at the Anglican church, and never did a Miss America have such godfathers: General Phillips and the Hessians, General von Knyphausen, and Colonel Wurmb.

The remaining months of spring 1780 were spent in the pleasant social activities of the city, but as summer arrived and the weather grew warmer, pestilence began to sweep New York. Sewage had been dumped on the ice all winter and now that the rivers were thawing, the muck backed up into the city's canals and streams, spreading every imaginable disease. Miss America was inoculated against smallpox and nearly died. The baron and his oldest daughter, Augusta, along with twenty other members of the household, fell ill with the malignant fever. As usual, Fritschen remained healthy, though she was pushed to the limits of her endurance in tending the sick. She wrote:

> Out of thirty persons of whom our family consisted, ten only escaped the disease. It is astonishing how much the frail human creature can endure; and I am amazed that I survived such hard trials. I rejoice to think that I had it in my power to be useful to those who are dearest to me, and that, without my exertions, I might have lost those who now contribute so much to my felicity. At length all my patients were cured.

In July the American general, Benjamin Lincoln, was captured by Clinton at Charleston, South Carolina. The Americans were anxious to get Lincoln back and entered into negotiations for his exchange. They must have wanted him very badly, for on October 31 he was traded for both Phillips and von Riedesel. Fritschen stayed in New York throughout the winter of 1781 while the baron took command of the Long Island garrison, headquartered at Brooklyn. In the spring, the baron secured a small farmhouse directly across the river from New York where he installed his family.

The von Riedesels remained in Brooklyn until July; the post was a difficult one, however, and the baron's health improved very little during this time. "Notwithstanding the loneliness of our situation," the baroness wrote, "we might have lived agreeably, had we not often been disturbed by the Americans as soon as the river was thawed. They frequently attempted surprises. . . . " A Major Maybaum was actually carried away from his bed one night, and the baron was afraid that he would be next. Vowing that he would never be taken prisoner again, the baron and his wife took turns standing guard each night; but as a result he got so little sleep that it merely aggravated his condition. Doctors advised that he leave the "foul climate" of Long Island, but in the present situation he could not ask for either a transfer or a furlough.

The securing of Long Island became increasingly difficult, not because of attack from the outside, but because, as General von Riedesel reported, "rebels [on the island] outnumbered Loyalists ten to one." Constant raids and dissension wore nerves thin and there seemed to be no practical way of bringing the populace under control. Anxious to leave, the baron now thought of his Brunswick regiments left behind in Canada years before. He appealed to Clinton to allow him to visit them, and in July the British commandant finally consented. The von Riedesels were to sail to Quebec, but not for a visit; the baron had been placed in command of all the German troops in Canada.

Of course the von Riedesels were glad at the prospect of rejoining their countrymen once again, and there was no sorrow at leaving behind the untenable military situation on Long Island. Since they had made several close friends among the British and American Loyalists in New York, many sad farewells were made.

Fritschen was no profiteer, so she returned all the fine furnishings that had been provided them by the British, though General Clinton said that they may as well keep them since it was "rebel furniture." When all their belongings were finally packed on board the ship that was to take them to Canada, there was far less than what they had started with years before.

The baroness's exultation at their return to a pleasant and orderly life in Canada was quickly overshadowed by the perils of the journey itself. Their ship was the smallest and worst-conditioned of the whole convoy in which they sailed, and it was so slow that they constantly lagged behind, thereby exposing themselves to the danger of American privateers. There were so many squalls and the ship leaked so badly that even Fritschen was pressed into service at the pumps. Food was scarce on board and the baron demanded that they be put ashore nightly so that provisions could be found for his family.

Somehow the little ship managed to reach the mouth of the St. Lawrence, but when they dropped anchor it came unfastened from its chain. With the boat drifting helplessly about, the baron could stand this show of incompetence no longer and insisted that he and his family be put ashore. Horses were purchased, and they set off along the river for Quebec.

Passing through the countryside, the baroness noted the pretty whitewashed houses and the little towns composed entirely of a single family. "They call themselves 'habitans,' " she wrote, "not peasants [because] the space around each [original] house is successively filled up by the settlements, which the young people on their marriages make around their parents." Other curiosities of the region came to Fritschen's attention—she described the "ice cellars" dug beneath the houses where food was preserved, even in the summer; the strange method of winter fishing where fish were caught through holes chopped in the ice; and the delicious "liquor" that was made from boiling the sap of the maple tree. "The Canadians are hospitable and cheerful," she wrote, "they sing and smoke the whole day."

The baron established his headquarters at Sorel, between Three Rivers and Montreal, and built a large two-story house for his family. A sizeable garden was attached where the von Riedesels grew all their own vegetables and fruits, and one of those curious "ice cellars" was dug in the basement.

By now the baron's health had improved considerably, owing probably to the crisp Canadian weather and the cleanliness and order of their surroundings. He had arrived in Quebec with a plan for conquering the American Patriots once and for all, and threw all his energies into putting it in effect. He and Clinton agreed that an attack should be launched toward the Ohio, while three or four well-fortified places were established on the coast from where the countryside could be harassed, thereby breaking the rebels' will to fight. The baron was sure that such fortifications would be impregnable because the Americans were incapable of making formal sieges against entrenched positions. In accordance with this plan, Cornwallis was sent to Yorktown, Virginia, to establish one of these "well-fortified places." In early November 1781 General von Riedesel learned of Lord Cornwallis's defeat at the hands of those same Patriots who were not adept at making sieges.

With the Battle of Yorktown, the war effectively came to an end, though the formal peace treaty would not be signed until the fall of 1783. There would be no more battles for General von Riedesel and the Brunswickers, just another year and a half of mechanical preparations for campaigns that everyone knew would not occur. This time passed quietly for the von Riedesels. Life at Sorel was not exciting, but there were frequent trips to Quebec and Montreal, and frequent visits from the officers of the garrison who were extremely fond of their baroness.

During this time Fritschen often accompanied her husband on his visits with their Indian allies, and she took the time to record a number of incidents. A German named Hansel, who had been raised by the Indians, arrived one day with his wife, whom he presented to the general. Fritschen recorded the exchange: " 'Hear! I love my wife,' said Hansel, 'but I love thee also: in proof of which I give her to thee!' Mr. de Riedesel replied, 'I thank thee and acknowledge thy attachment, but I have a wife whom I also love, and beg thee to keep thy own.' The man seemed distressed and almost offended at this refusal, and he could hardly be persuaded to carry his wife back, who, as having seen her afterwards, I can attest was very pretty." On another occasion she relates a story about "a certain Johnson" who became a rich man by playing on the great significance that Indians attached to dreams. It seems that the Indians would come to see him and mention that they had dreamed that Johnson had given them rum and tobacco, whereupon Johnson would prove them right by giving them their favorite delicacies. This went on for quite awhile and, of course, the dreams became more frequent, until one day Johnson went to tell the Indians,

> that he had, also, had a dream: that in return for the kindness and hospitality he had shown them, they had granted him a large tract of land, which he described. "Have you really dreamt that?" they exclaimed with countenances expressive of terror; and having said this they went into deliberation; at the conclusion of which they returned to him, and said, "Brother Johnson, we give thee that tract of land—but never dream any more."

The Indians were not only a source of amusement to the baroness;

they were often guests at her table, and she noted their civility and noble bearing. She did write that they were faithful allies only in victory, though she ascribes their unwillingness to fight when the tables were turned, to their sensible fear of capture and death. After all, they were not Germans. In general, she seems to have been highly impressed by these "savages."

In November 1782 Fritschen gave birth to another child, but again the von Riedesels' hopes for a son were frustrated. The little girl, whom they named Canada, died within five months, and the baroness ordered "an inscription engraved upon her tomb, to save it from any profanation which it might suffer, on the score of our religious principles, from some zealous Canadian Catholic." The von Riedesels, of course, were Lutherans.

There was great sorrow at this loss, probably more than at the death of previous children, for now it was compounded by the uselessness of their position in Canada and their growing homesickness. The baroness was being gallant when she wrote that they would have been "glad to remain longer in Canada, for the climate proved favourable to our children; and we had many friends and our situation was altogether agreeable," for she quickly added, "I was anxious to see my family again."

By July 1783 preliminary peace negotiations were under way in Paris, and the baron was finally recalled. In the middle of August the von Riedesels and the Brunswick regiments set sail for England, and on October 8 received heroes' welcomes as they marched back into their beloved town of Wolfenbuttel. Out of 4,000 Brunswickers who came to America, only 2,800 returned. Of the seventy-seven women who had marched out of town that day in 1776, thirteen had either died or deserted in America. At the age of thirty-eight, Fritschen was grateful to be home; she knew how often she had come close to being one of the casualties.

In Brunswick the baroness became noted for her kindness to visiting Americans. She had been spat upon by those outrageous Patriots in the streets of Boston, and she vowed that the insults would not be repaid in kind.

Fritschen forgot little of those six fantastic years in America, and some time later she published a family edition of her memoirs. It became so popular among the German aristocracy that a public edition was soon gotten out which was more or less accurately translated into English. American "scholars" took great liberties with it, and in several hurriedly thrown-together postwar histories, descriptions of the baroness range from a "small Dresden china figure" to "Amazonian." The baroness never saw any of these books, but it is doubtful that the discrepancies would have bothered her much. She was secure and self-assured in her own recollections of her experiences, and she was not one to bear grudges—even against her former enemies. Life was simply a matter of duty, which had to be performed with alacrity and good will, and most important was duty to one's family. The male heir, Georg Karl, was finally born in Brunswick in 1785.

11

Margaret Shippen Arnold

THE PARTY was almost over, and the majority of the pleasantly tired guests had gone out into the wintry night. The servants clattered dishes out of the ballroom, and the orchestra wearily played a few last tunes for the benefit of the new American hero and his constant companion of that evening. Pretty young Margaret Shippen (whom everyone called Peggy) sat basking in the conversational warmth of the Eagle of Saratoga, whose military leadership and valor at the battle of Saratoga had catapulted him to fame. But Benedict Arnold was losing another battle at his own party. He was indeed a willing victim of the wiles and charm of teenaged Peggy Shippen, whose social prowess and discreet charm belied her years. Aside from the usual attraction a young woman would feel toward an officer and a war hero, the maturity of Arnold—who was nearly twice Peggy's age—enhanced the general in her wily blue eyes. Like Lord Byron, he had a pronounced limp which, rather than putting women off, served to make their hearts flutter even more. It mattered little to Peggy that she could not dance with her escort that night. She was the companion of the star of the ball, and all the other women knew it and envied her.

Eighteenth-century warfare being the decorous institution it was, a person attending Arnold's party that night in 1778 would have had reason to doubt that a war was going on at all. If anything, Philadelphia's social gaiety flourished even more, due to the profusion of eligible young men in both the British and American occupations and the large number of society women who resided in the city. Arnold, appointed military governor of Philadelphia in June 1778, sought in Philadelphia to reward himself and his officers for their privations and injuries in the American cause, with a brilliant social life.

And so another party soon followed this one, and many more came after. The resultant gaiety only served to increase the general's ardor toward Peggy Shippen. He finally proposed, but Peggy's father, Edward Shippen, refused him because of the age discrepancy. Peggy continued, however, to welcome Arnold's attentions. In fact, the economic disaster which had consumed the once significant Shippen fortunes made Arnold seem a likely candidate for Peggy's hand, since his new wealth would permit Peggy to live in the style to which she had been accustomed.

Arnold's fortunes not only interested his prospective bride and father-in-law but also the colonial government as well. He was even put under Congressional scrutiny and faced court-martial for allegedly using his rank and reputation for illegal war profiteering. As a matter of fact, Arnold had, so far, done little more than many of his fellow officers, who amassed considerable financial means by peddling their influence. Joseph Reed, president of the Supreme Executive Council of Pennsylvania, suspected Arnold of using public property for personal ends. Lacking evidence, Congress almost dropped charges against the Saratoga hero, but Reed and the Philadelphia Council goaded Congress into passing the matter on to a military court-martial.

Arnold's difficulty served only to heighten his love for Peggy, who provided unflagging support for him throughout the ordeal of accusation and counteraccusation. Mrs. Robert Morris wrote that "Cupid has given our little general a more mortal wound than all the host of Britons could. . . . Miss Peggy Shippen is the fair one." And on April 8, 1779, Benedict Arnold and Peggy Shippen were wed. Although their courtship had been marked by great luxury, the wedding was small and simple. Arnold had paid for the courtship, but Edward Shippen paid for the wedding with the meager resources left from a great prewar fortune. Arnold was required to lean on a soldier as he spoke his wedding vows, since his wounded leg continued to cause him great pain.

From the time of the wedding there was considerable speculation as to the couple's treasonable activities. Undoubtedly part of this suspicion arose from the fact that Peggy's family was split in its loyalty to the colonial cause. The Shippens were a prominent old family in Philadelphia and Margaret's father was a London-educated attorney. Edward's active civic life in Pennsylvania had included his serving as judge of the Vice-Admiralty Court, town clerk, member and clerk of the Common Council and Protonotary

of the Supreme Court of Pennsylvania. Although politically sophisticated and sensible in judgment, Shippen was unoriginal and
cautious in both business and the law. With the passage of the
Stamp Act in 1765, Shippen gave up his business, since obedience
would expose him to local harassment and disobedience would lead
to royal persecution. When the hated act was repealed in 1766,
Shippen returned to business and held parties in honor of King
George. At the time even hotheads were likely to theorize that it was
a corrupt government and not an evil king who used America so
badly. Shippen continued to vacillate in fear of both royal preroga-
tives and colonial street mobs, and he steered a middle course as
carefully as he could. His timidity was a far cry from the activity of
his father, who became chairman of the Lancaster, Pennsylvania,
Committee of Safety.

Shippen's noncommital attitude finally failed. Responding to a
series of threats to his family's safety, at times Edward moved them
away from the glitter and excitement of Philadelphia. When the
guns sounded on the horizon, the family quickly removed to their
country residence. When rural suspicions against supposed Loyalists were excited, the Shippens returned to Philadelphia. Then
persecutions of Loyalists began again in Philadelphia, and the
Shippens repaired to a different farm. Lists of so-called Loyalists
slated for attention included the entire Shippen family, despite
Edward's cautious efforts to maintain a reputation of neutrality.

It was unsafe for the friends and relatives of the Shippens to visit
them in their various country retreats. Peggy's cousin with her
children had been attacked by a colonial militia company whose
leaders had resented the elegance of her carriage. Such incidents
discouraged other visitors. The isolation of the very social Shippen
girls in country exile must have been felt acutely.

Shippen traveled almost daily to the Patriot-held city of Philadelphia to make the family home appear occupied and, therefore, a less
likely candidate for the quartering of troops. Any person who
traveled without a permit was subject to arrest as a spy; consequent-
ly, Shippen was placed on house arrest on his farm. The sentence
eventually was revoked, and at about the same time, the Shippens
and the British arrived in Philadelphia.

The capture of the city by the British resulted in social elegance
unparalleled before the Revolution. Although Shippen declined the
jobs offered him by the conquerers, he allowed his daughters to
engage in the social festivities that abounded in the city. Shippen's

main worry then shifted to his daughters' maintaining their virtue. He had little reason to worry. Although many illegitimate children were fathered during the occupation, few of the mothers were well-connected girls.

Peggy was one of the most popular young women. Lord Rawdon considered her the handsomest woman he had seen in America, and Captain A. S. Hammond of the H. M. S. *Roebuck* remembered, "We were all in love with her." Major John André also developed an interest in Peggy, but it was another Peggy, Peggy Chew, who actually won André's heart. The elegant Miss Shippen did manage, however, to save a lock of André's hair until the day she died. Such locks were considered tokens of friendship in the eighteenth century. André also painted a portrait of Peggy. Speculation about any romantic attachment between André and Peggy remains merely that. No evidence exists to ascertain the extent of their affection, since the Shippen family destroyed his letters and any other evidence linking the two.

The Shippen girls were not displeased with the British capture of their city since life became a long series of parties and balls. The social high point of the British occupation of Philadelphia was the Meschianza, an extravagant Turkish ball given on May 18, 1778. It was meant to be a spectacular send-off for General Howe, who had been recalled to England for a job not well done. The Meschianza was produced, directed, and choreographed by Major André. The soldier-artist saw no incongruity in combining a medieval jousting tournament with Turkish decorations. The Shippen sisters were scheduled to act as the ladies of the knights. Whether Peggy and her sisters actually did participate in the event cannot be proven. The Shippen family claims that Edward refused to allow his daughters to attend the affair, since the very idea of such a send-off for General Howe aroused the ire of local Patriots. Other evidence, such as the appearance of the Shippen girls' names on the printed guest list, indicates that they probably were there. It is perhaps also significant that Peggy wore her Meschianza costume for André's portrait of her.

A month later Arnold took over Philadelphia and, not long after, Peggy Shippen's heart. The thirty-six-year-old war hero found it in his heart to write Peggy of his burning desire for her:

> Till then; all nature smiles in vain, for you alone, heard, felt, and seen possess my every thought, fill every sense, and pant in every vein.

Arnold must have been pleased with the tone and style of letters such as this, since he had already used them in his futile pursuit of Betsy Deblois of Boston.

Peggy made Arnold forget Betsy quite handily. However, his association with the Shippen family increased the disaffection his shady military/business interests had brought him. Because of Edward Shippen's vacillation between the English and American sides, many had branded him a Loyalist. No doubt his daughter's prolonged social affiliations with outright Loyalists had served to heighten suspicions about the Shippen family's fidelity to the colonial cause. Passionate revolutionaries counted it treason to befriend suspected Loyalists. Efforts against Arnold may have been motivated partly by Peggy's insulting behavior toward Joseph Reed's wife.

The couple began actively to consider treason about the time of their marriage. Peggy's participation in the treasonous events which followed have inspired much historical debate. At this time in the late 1770s, the Arnolds had every reason to believe that loyalty to the revolutionary cause would be unprofitable. Even more distressing, Arnold felt he had been singled out for punishment in the court-martial proceedings against him. Arnold was stung by the fact that General Washington, bound to neutrality by both politics and personal conviction, did not come to his aid. Washington did, however, appoint Arnold to the command of West Point, which was an invalid regiment. Although the command was not the most glamorous of appointments, it served as an important bartering item for Arnold, who soon promised to surrender it to the British. The capture of West Point would enable the British to split the colonies in two and pave the way for a British victory.

Even before Washington signed his orders, Arnold had offered the fort to the British. He pressed for specific commitments to reward him for service and to repay losses if the plan failed. General Clinton, head of British forces, offered £500 for previous intelligence and £20,000 for capture of West Point with 3,000 men. André further encouraged the Arnolds by telling Peggy that more could be arranged for when Arnold and André met under a flag of truce. Peggy joined her husband at West Point to tell him of André's offer and so that Arnold could spend more time with their son Edward.

She had resided at West Point less than a month when Major André was captured, thus exposing Arnold's involvement in the West Point plot. Once again historical accounts differ as to the degree of Peggy's involvement in her husband's affairs, but it seems likely that she did play an important role in discovering means by which her husband could communicate with ranking British officers. A crockery dealer, Joseph Stansbury, carried Arnold's messages through the British lines to General Henry Clinton.

The Americans who had discovered André sent one letter to Washington explaining Arnold's participation in the crime and another letter to Arnold outlining the evidence against him. Perhaps the motive behind the letter to Arnold was to leave him alone with his gun, since it was not known that escape by sea was available to him.

Immediately after Arnold and Peggy received the letter, his aide announced that Washington was a short distance away. Arnold took off for a nearby British ship, leaving his wife alone in the house when Washington arrived. Her hysteria was diagnosed as wounded, innocent patriotism. Washington and all his aides expressed pity for the unfortunate and betrayed woman who, with her child, was abandoned by a traitor. Alexander Hamilton wrote this account of the scene:

> One moment she raved, another she melted into tears. Sometimes she pressed her infant to her bosom and lamented its fate occasioned by the imprudence of its father, in a manner that would have pierced insensibility itself. All the sweetness of beauty, all the loveliness of innocence, all the tenderness of a wife, and all the fondness of a mother showed themselves in her appearance and conduct. . . . It was the most affecting scene I ever was witness to. Could I forgive Arnold for sacrificing his honor, reputation, and duty, I could not forgive him for acting a part that must have forfeited the esteem of so fine a woman.

Peggy's safety depended on her playing the part of innocence so well that no official would even think of the possibility that she might share her husband's guilt. General Washington, his officers, and a physician agreed on the cause of her hysteria, and Washington wrote a pass to guarantee safe conduct back to her family in Philadelphia.

Margaret Shippen Arnold met in Philadelphia the violent hatred reserved for traitors to the cause of nationalist struggle. Whereas Washington's officer corps could not believe a frail woman in hysterics capable of treason, the people of Philadelphia were suspicious of a woman so recently considered a prominent Loyalist. Edward Shippen personally took charge of the effort to down

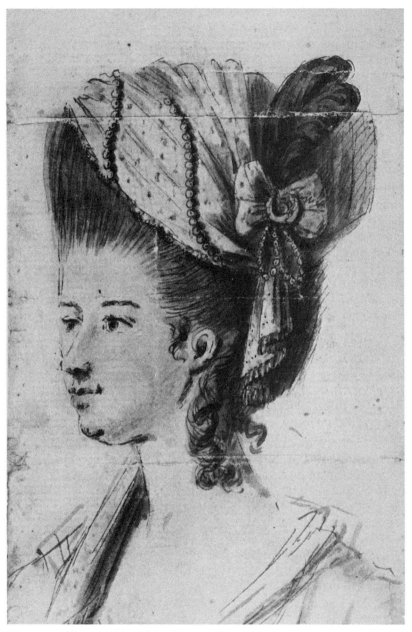

Margaret Shippen Arnold (Portrait by Major John André)
Courtesy, The Historical Society of Pennsylvania

accusations against his daughter. Nevertheless, search warrants obtained all the Arnolds' papers which had not been destroyed. Found among the papers was evidence to prove that Arnold had been guilty of the charges of corrupt commerce. A nasty letter written after a social event put the sweetness of Peggy's personality under suspicion and angered the subjects. Seizing on a letter André had written from New York in which he offered Peggy millinery service, the *Pennsylvania Packet* argued that the document disproved "the fallacious and dangerous sentiments so frequently avowed in this city that female opinions are of no consequence in public matters." Although at one point Peggy sought to remain in Philadelphia and offered to show Arnold's letters and papers to his enemies, she finally was exiled to her husband's side. Arnold allowed his wife to play the injured party the rest of her life.

However, this picture of the wife brutally deceived, not in love but in politics, clashes dramatically with her own acknowledgment of complicity in her husband's crimes. Apparently, Peggy confided her part in her husband's treason to the widow of a British officer with whom she stayed on her return from West Point in 1780. That widow, Mrs. Theodosia Prevost, later married Aaron Burr, from whom the story came long after both the Arnolds were dead. Because of the late emergence of this version of Peggy's sympathies, and because of the widespread conviction of her innocence, this piece of evidence often has been discounted. Certainly a contributing factor to the belief in her innocence arose from the popular mythology about female limitations. Undoubtedly, many of those who defended Peggy were doing so from the perspective that a woman simply was incapable of such high-level deception. However, the opening of the papers of Henry Clinton, who masterminded Arnold's espionage activities, indicate that Peggy was awarded £350 "for her services, which were very meritorious." This evidence of substantial payment to Peggy proved what before had merely been speculation.

After she and her little son Edward were forced to leave Pennsylvania, Peggy joined her husband in New York. Their reunion was short-lived, however, as Arnold soon led a British attack in Virginia. But as British defeat in the war became imminent, the Arnolds sailed for England and what Peggy regarded as safety. There two daughters and another son were born to them. Only one of the daughters survived.

Peggy and Arnold joined the London social scene with the grace and flair they had exhibited in America. Peggy was especially sought after because of her charm and beauty. However, she had to bear many difficulties, as a letter to her father indicates:

> I assure you, my dear Papa, I find it necessary to summon all my philosophy to my aid to support myself under my present situation.
>
> Separated from, and anxious for the fate of the best of husbands, torn from almost everybody that is dear to me, harassed with a troublesome and expensive lawsuit, having all the General's business to transact, and feeling that I am in a strange country, without a creature near me that is really interested in my fate, you will not wonder if I am unhappy.

Arnold longed to be placed in active combat by the British government, but he saw little military action the rest of his life. Instead, he turned to business again, engaging in trade primarily with the West Indies. His business interests required some trips to Canada, where he was occasionally accompanied by Peggy and their children. Only once did Peggy return to America, when the ill health of her mother prompted her to sail from the social safety of England to her hometown of Philadelphia. Although Peggy thought that anti-Arnold feeling would surely have diminished dramatically, she was wrong. Most Philadelphians treated her cooly, regarding her as a traitor to the American cause.

Peggy returned to London dismayed but seemed able to forget her unhappiness by plunging into the social activities that she and her husband had always loved.

In June 1801 Benedict Arnold died with his wife by his side. A family friend recorded the scene:

> She evinces upon this occasion, as you know she has done on many trying ones before, that fortitude and resignation, which a superior and well-regulated mind only is capable of exerting.

Peggy had to deal not only with her grief over the loss of her adored husband but also with considerable debts accumulated during Arnold's business ventures. Provided by Parliament with pensions for herself and her children, and with help from her father, Peggy managed to pay all her dead husband's debts. In one of her letters, she wrote about the many sacrifices she had been forced to make:

I have been under the necessity of parting with my furniture, wine and many other comforts provided for me by the indulgent hand of affection; and have by these sacrifices paid all the ascertained debts, within a few hundred pounds.

Three years after her husband's death on August 24, 1804, Peggy Shippen Arnold, a social sensation even in middle age, died in London at the age of forty.

PART IV

Women on Their Own

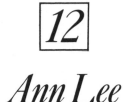

Ann Lee

T HE THREE COMMISSIONERS for detecting and defeating conspira-
cies in the state of New York were troubled by the little group of
radicals living in the swampy wilderness beyond the city of Albany.
Matthew Adgate, the justice of the peace for an area east of the river
town, had informed the investigators that some of the group were,
quite likely, British spies or were, at least, conspiring to aid the
enemy.

Adgate had arrested three of the Shakers while they were driving
sheep from their farms in New Lebanon, near where the state
bordered on Massachusetts, to the Shaker colony north of Albany,
in the Indian district called Niskeyuna. The Shakers had a "disaffection to the American Cause," the justice told the commissioners,
charging that the men were most likely trying to take the sheep "to
the Enemy or at least bring them so near the Frontiers that the
enemy may with safety take them."

The commissioners were especially concerned about Albany and
its environs, though their task of ferreting out British and Loyalist
plots had led them to hold sessions throughout the state. Less than
three years had passed since the British had attempted to march
down from Canada and capture Albany, thus separating New York
from New England. Burgoyne had been turned back at Saratoga.
After a period of relative quiet, the volatile Iroquois Indians, allies of
the redcoats, had begun again to make terrifying forays into the area
northwest of Albany.

The commissioners jailed the three men, although the farmers
had proved their intentions were not treasonous. They were only
driving their sheep to Niskeyuna because the colony was in great
need of provisions to feed the numbers who were flocking to Mother

Ann Lee, the colony's founder, to be saved. But the commissioners distrusted the activity—there *was* a war going on—and were especially concerned since Mother Lee, as well as several other Shakers, were British. The eccentric woman may only have been proselytizing for converts out there in the swamps, but the commissioners could not be sure. Adgate told them that many of the group were avowed Loyalists, but the commissioners heard these Shaker farmers heatedly deny the authority of their investigations, and, indeed, all civil authority.

One of the men, David Darrow, scarred from service in the war, told the commission that he was through with warfare since the Shakers preached pacifism, and that he would "not in any instance . . . abide by the Laws of the State." Joseph Meacham, one of Ann Lee's most recent converts, declared that he, too, had a "determined Resolution never to take up arms and to dissuade others from doing the same."

If the act of driving sheep to the colony was not treasonous, such talk was! The commissioners ruled that the principles of the men were "highly pernicious and of destructive tendency to the Freedom and Independence of the United States of America," and promptly locked up Darrow and the two farmers, letting Meacham and another witness return to Niskeyuna with the ominous news.

The arrests were only the first in a series of harassments the Shakers were to suffer during the War of Independence. The time called for unquestioning loyalty to the cause, especially now at the turn of the decade when the Americans seemed to be facing, at the very best, a stalemate in the war. The situation around Albany was tense and had been for years. More than a score of citizens from the area had gone over to the British side.

Under such circumstances, no group of people could have appeared more suspect than the Shakers. They were, according to conventional opinion, bizarre fanatics—people who during their wild church services could behave with ungodly abandon, undergo fits of "shaking," and speak in tongues. Their ideas seemed extremely strange—the Shakers preached celibacy, and Mother Ann Lee, seemingly a blasphemer, had claimed to be a reincarnation of Christ. Many were sure she was possessed by the devil and practiced witchcraft.

The tiny band of Shakers was disturbing, too, because they had been successful in attracting American converts, not only poor, uneducated itinerants, but also men and women of some substance as well. One of their leaders was a John Hocknell, a propertied Englishman. American converts included Meacham, who had been a lay preacher; Samuel Johnson, a Yale graduate who joined the Shakers with his wife; Darrow, the brother of a prosperous New York farmer; and Daniel Goodrich, the son of a deacon in the Baptist Church. Why were such upstanding citizens giving up their communities, their livelihoods and reputations to live out in the wilderness? Were they trying to avoid the war? Were they, in being sympathetic to British Shakers, part of a British plot?

The fact that all in the group were actively proselytizing for members—and actively espousing conscientious objection—led the commissioners to arrest Mother Ann Lee along with five other Shaker leaders in late July 1780. The imprisonment of the leader did not mark her first stay in jail, only her first in America—the land where, the English Shakers had seen in revelation, there was a "chosen people" who would accept Mother Lee's gospel and establish, quite literally, a heaven on earth.

When she stood before the commissioners, Ann Lee was approaching her middle forties, and from her appearance she seemed to be anything but a witch. She was, perhaps, a little shorter than most women, rather thickset, and just a little plain. If the commissioners had heard of the wild utterances and prophecies of the woman, she gave no evidence of such when they examined her. If anything, she appeared cooly dignified, with her simple manners and mild bearing, as she told of her belief in both peace and the American cause.

The Shakers had had a vision of founding a church in America, she told the commissioners, and she had herself foreseen the colonial war and the ultimate American victory. These events, she testified, were an act of Providence which would lead to the millennium in America.

The commissioners distrusted the woman, of course. Too many incredible stories were circulating throughout the region to allow them to give credence to her simple testimony. And how could she believe in the American cause and yet counsel pacifism? For the commissioners, as for Americans in general, the war was concerned with political and economic freedoms and liberties and not religious issues. Certainly and most decidedly, it was not a war which would establish the kingdom of God in America! With material freedoms at stake, the cause was now a military affair. Such apocalyptic preachings as performed by Ann Lee in the wilderness seemed threatening.

Twice she had been imprisoned before in England at the beginning of her extraordinary career as a religious leader. In 1772 she spent a month in jail at Manchester with her father and a handful of others for the crime of "breaking the Sabbath" and for assault on some of the twenty-four officers who had come to quiet down the noisome Shaker meetings. A year later, she was arrested again for "disturbing the Congregation in the old church" at Manchester. Unable to pay the twenty-pound fine, she was locked up for over two weeks.

It was this imprisonment which confirmed her natural election as leader of the Shakers in England. While being kept in a cell so small she couldn't stand, starved and given nothing to drink, she had had a vision, a "grand vision of the very transgression of the first man and woman in the Garden of Eden, the cause wherein all mankind was lost and separated from God." In the vision Christ appeared to her—this revelation made her his special instrument. "It is not I that speak," she told the Shakers after the ordeal, "it is Christ who dwells in me."

This messianic vision and her "call" to America, which was soon to follow, firmly established her leadership of the Shakers. The group would become important in America, contributing a set of ideas and a pattern of life which added substantial richness to the mosaic of American cultural diversity. Their evolving emphasis on fellowship and community, and their colorful heritage of songs, dances, art, architecture, and daily rituals, all celebrated a simple democratic faith. After their early years of crisis in America, they would prove themselves to be among the most successful of voluntary societies.

The group was baptized twice, in England and in America, and Ann Lee was the central figure in both events. Her role was as enormous and important as her background was tawdry and obscure. Born the second of eight children to a poor blacksmith who died when Ann was in her teens, the woman who was to become a major religious mystic had no education other than that provided by work in the bleak mills of Manchester.

From the age of four, she worked in a mill manufacturing cotton and later as a cutter of hatters' fur. Such mills were, for many, the "perfect image of hell." She labored in this cruel environment like thousands of other Manchester factory girls who—in the words of one observer of the time—toiled "like slaves living under a mortal fear of losing their jobs . . . driven to perform work so unflagging and demanding that a grown man . . . would not be able to bear up under the strain."

Her home life was equally grim. She returned from work to her home on Toad Lane, a grimy street occupied almost solely by blacksmiths and publicans, to find virtually no room for herself in the crowded house. She developed at a very young age a heightened sense of the debauched nature of such conditions, which were typical of the times and, according to one health report, a "baptism in infamy" for the children. The close quarters had exposed Ann to acts she considered vile and gruesome and violent. When she was quite young, she had chastised her mother several times for making love with her father. Enraged, her father had threatened her each time and tried to whip her.

Her parents were religious people and Ann was to follow them in their intensity, if not, ultimately, in their specific beliefs. Distraught by the degradation of her life, she had tried several times to break free. At the age of twenty, she went to work as a cook in a public infirmary, an occupation that was later to account for charges by her enemies that she had been incarcerated in a madhouse. Two years later at a turning point in her life, she joined a society of radical religious dissenters who practiced their faith in the drab industrial town of Bolton on-the-Moors.

The group was led by James and Jane Wardley, two tailors from Bolton. They had been Quakers, members of the Society of Friends, but had come under the influence of radical French Calvinism through a sect called the Camisards, and had established their own church. During this time of the Industrial Revolution, England was undergoing a period of disturbing popular unrest which was soon to manifest itself in the intense activities of the Luddites, a movement of thousands who protested industrialism by ransacking factories and destroying machinery. Already the great consternation of the times was evident in the rise of popular evangelical movements, and the Wardleys spearheaded one such crusade.

They developed a series of rituals—trances, fasts, fits of shaking, a belief in signs and revelations, and prophesying the coming of the end of the world and the second coming of Christ—that raised to a new level of energy the practices of their "quaking" past. Because of their origins and rituals, followers became known as the "Shaking Quakers." They provided a strong counter to the piety and decorum of the establishment faith, Anglicanism, and a more intense involvement by participants than that practiced in such a sect as Quakerism.

The activities were important to Ann; they offered a way for her to work off her tensions and communicate the terrible strains of her existence. She officially remained a member of the Anglican Church until sometime after her marriage in 1762 to a blacksmith named Abraham Standerin. Abraham worked with Ann's father, and though she did not want to marry, her parents forced the union.

The next years were decisive ones for her commitment to and modification of the Wardleys' faith. From childhood on, she had been disgusted by sexuality, and the marriage was excruciatingly painful for her. She bore four children in nearly successive years, three of whom died in infancy, the other living only to the age of six. Her last childbirth had been torture, the delivery by forceps nearly killing her.

The births were—and she was grotesquely accurate in her description—violations of her body, and she swore off sex altogether. She came to see the deaths of her children as judgments by God on her "concupiscence" and avoided sharing her bed with Abraham "as if it were made of embers."

It was a period of great psychological torment, and undoubtedly helped give rise to the overwhelming tendency toward exaggeration which became her most consistent practice as a Shaker leader. So anguished was she at the time, she later reported, that "bloody sweat" would pour through her skin. When she would wring her hands, blood "gushed from under her nails," and the tears she cried flowed so hotly down her cheeks that they "cleaved off" her skin.

She screamed throughout the night and rocked in her bed in so agitated a manner that Abraham was "glad to leave it." Finally she began to deny herself "every gratification of a carnal nature;" she ate only those things which were "mean and poor" so that she "might hunger for nothing but God."

She gave herself up totally to the Wardleys. Her childhood and adolescence had been wretched; she could not tolerate the pattern to continue into adulthood. Abraham was so exasperated that he complained to Anglican church authorities about her, but the great distress caused by the childbirths held sway. Her needs were evident in the testimony she made when she dedicated herself irrevocably to God. "My soul broke forth to God," she said, "which I felt as sensibly as ever a woman did a child, when she was delivered of it."

Her last child had died in October 1767, an event that marked her increasing activity with the Wardleys and the development of a total conviction of her mission in life. She saw her own suffering as a sign of the universal struggle of all men and women, with the deaths of her children representing to her "the deplorable loss of the human race."

By the late 1760s the Wardleys had become known and notorious throughout the region. Their membership had grown, and among the new converts were some wealthy men whose resources allowed the group to expand their activities. As the Shakers grew, however, so grew their opposition. Popularly they were charged with heresy and witchcraft, and Ann herself was called before a council of ministers to testify about her faith. She told her companions that she had been threatened with branding of her body and burning of her tongue, but that she had spoken in tongues and the ministers, marveling at the feat, had released her.

With each charge of fanaticism and attempt at suppression, the Shakers grew more adamant in their beliefs. Ann herself contributed to dozens of stories about persecutions of the group, telling many times of being stoned and beaten by mobs. By the time she had spent her weeks in prison for refusing to pay her fine for breaking up a gathering of worshippers at an Anglican church, she had developed a firm persecution complex that justified the avid, even feverish, proselytizing by the group.

It was perhaps a decrease in the persecution that led Ann to take her followers across the sea to America. She had become—after her imprisonment—"Mother" Ann Lee, taking the title and the leadership that had belonged to Jane Wardley. Her rise was coincident with a decision by authorities not to harass the Shakers as long as they made no outrageous displays of themselves in the streets. The Shakers relied on the publicity of persecution to attract new members, but with this decision of government leaders the Shakers experienced no new membership growth.

Ann Lee arrived in New York with eight of her followers in early August 1774. With her was James Whittaker, a passionate Shaker who had seen the church in America appear in a vision of a large tree whose leaves "shone with brightness, as it made it appear a burning torch." The little band arrived with no church to greet them, but according to Shaker testimonies, Ann immediately led the group to a nearby home. There she told the mistress of the household named Cunningham, "I am commissioned of the Almighty God to preach the everlasting Gospel to America, and an Angel commanded me to come to this house, and to make a home for me and my people."

The woman took the Shakers in, and Ann was soon spending her first weeks in America as a domestic in the Cunningham house. Other Shakers found similar kinds of employment and waited for a sign that would lead them to found a church. They were sure such a sign would come, for on the voyage they had been assured of their mission when their ship—in a seemingly miraculous manner—was saved from capsizing.

They lived frugally in New York until they heard of inexpensive land near Albany, and three of the members traveled up the Hudson to investigate. Ann and the others were left behind to keep working and to save money. The three quickly sent word that they might lease property from wealthy landowners, the Stuyvesants, in the Indian district past Albany, a swampy, wooded area known as Niskeyuna. The men worked for a time in Albany at such trades as blacksmithing and weaving, and within a year had both leased the land and begun to clear a portion of it for a crude wooden cabin.

Mother Ann visited Niskeyuna and approved of the activities, but she remained primarily in New York City to work at washing and ironing, earning money to support the venture in the wilderness. She stayed in New York too because her husband Abraham was there. He had accompanied Ann and the Shakers to America. Decidedly not a believer, he hoped to win Ann back, nevertheless. For her part, Ann hoped to convert Abraham to Shakerism and was committed personally to him, her last connection with her old identity.

The new land, however, led to no new relationship between the two. They lived only infrequently together, even though he was employed with Ann at the Cunningham household as a blacksmith. Abraham, increasingly frustrated, entered a state of debauchery that confirmed Ann's worst fears, not only about him but also about the universal condition of the degenerate. Though she nursed him back from ill health for a period of a year, even quitting her work to do so and thus denying herself her contribution to the colony at Niskeyuna, their marriage finally and officially broke up. Abraham, back in health, took up his degenerate ways, threatening that he would leave Ann to live with a loathsome prostitute he had brought by to exhibit, unless Ann changed her staunch practice of celibacy. Sickened, Ann refused, and the marriage of thirteen years ended.

Wholly alone now, with Abraham gone and her Shaker followers now living in the north, Ann spent most of the year of 1775 living in the crudest of circumstances in the city. She stayed in a tiny room without a bed or heat, its only furnishing being a coal stove. She even denied herself food so that she might give more to the group at Niskeyuna. Much of the time she sipped her dinner from a cruse of vinegar.

At Christmastime things brightened, for a wealthy Shaker bene-factor, John Hocknell, who had funded the first voyage, brought on his return to America both his wife and his monied brother-in-law, John Partington. His wife, Mary, would become Ann's constant companion. The infusion of both freshened spirits and new cash gave the group at Niskeyuna a great boost, and by March the colony was well enough established for Mother Ann to join the group permanently. Her departure from New York City had become a necessity, as it was apparent that the city would be a battleground in the war. The American General Washington had stationed 10,000 troops throughout Manhattan, and before the British General Howe sailed down from Nova Scotia and took Staten Island with his 25,000 men, Ann Lee had left for Niskeyuna.

The colony was to suffer for the next three years through sometimes dispiriting labor. Survival itself was the immediate problem. Some of the Shaker men continued to work at Albany while the remaining group of men and women stayed on their land at Niskeyuna, performing the pioneer chores of clearing and tilling the land, making the swampy area suitable for both habitation and cultivation. By 1779 the group was ecstatic over the building of a frame house, but it burned down shortly after its construction.

The difficulties hardened the Shaker faith, though there was not much material evidence to justify optimism. A missionary group, they had prepared to receive what they thought were the hundreds, perhaps thousands, that would convert. In three years, however, only one neighbor woman from this area populated by a few scattered settlements had joined them. Ann told her brother, " . . . the time is near at hand when they will come like doves." But they didn't come, and while living conditions in the colony im-proved, it seemed their mission might be failing. "O that the fishes of the sea and fowls of the air, and all things that have life, yea, all the trees of the forest and grass of the trees," Ann cried in the wilderness, "would pray to God for me!"

In the spring of 1779, Mother Ann began to have visions of converts coming to the settlement, and she ordered that the group put up stores of food for their arrival. Prescient or shrewd, she sensed that the religious revivals that were occurring throughout the region would benefit the colony. "We shall have company enough," she told her brother, and soon her sense proved correct.

The group had established itself at a fortuitous moment, for the entire region was undergoing the outbreak of religious fervor known as the Great Awakening. That frenzy had begun as early as the 1730s when Jonathan Edwards, minister at Northampton, Massachusetts, began his ardent preachings. Even now in the late 1770s, revivals were still common, and in June a particularly intense outbreak was occurring on the New York-Massachusetts border, not far from Albany. Situated primarily in New Lebanon, New York, but reaching into several adjacent towns, the fervid revival played itself out by fall, leaving its participants exhausted from their emotional outpourings of faith and depressed that there had been no manifestations of the Second Coming. By the next spring the revival seemed to be over; in despair the believers left the region.

However, two of the group journeying west from New Lebanon came upon the Shaker community at Niskeyuna. They were amazed and impressed by the colony and became convinced that Ann Lee was truly, as she testified, the risen Christ. They hurried back to New Lebanon anxious to spread the news that the meetings there had not been in vain, and that God had responded to them through the providential meeting with Mother Ann Lee.

The leader of the New Lebanon revival, Joseph Meacham, responded by sending out his chief lieutenant, Calvin Harlow, to investigate. Harlow returned exultant, completely under the sway of the charismatic woman, and the success of the Shakers was secure.

Meacham gathered up the remainder of the New Lebanon believers and quickly set out for Niskeyuna. He became the "first-born son"—the first prestigious American convert—and following him came the many who were to make Niskeyuna such a suspicious place in the eyes of the war-worried in Albany.

The jailing of Ann Lee and other Shaker leaders gave great publicity to the colony. As in England, the Shakers ultimately profited from this harassment which focused attention on their ideas and beliefs. The exposure given the group was tremendous. Not only were they able to attract followers who would camp outside the Albany jail to hear Ann and others preach through the bars, there was even pressure building from Albany's respectable citizenry to release the group. To many it seemed inconceivable that, during a war which was being fought over the issues of freedom and liberty, the government was persecuting a seemingly harmless religious sect.

There was pressure from both sides, however. The government feared what it thought was a pro-British group and worried that the Shakers might be providing a haven for those who, like Darrow, wanted to find refuge during a war they were sickened by. In an effort to break up the group, Ann Lee was banished down the Hudson in mid-August "for the purpose of being removed within the Enemy's Lines."

The Albany Commission had decided that Mother Ann should be sent to New York where a prisoner exchange could be worked out with the British. Whether the English rejected the plan—what did General Howe want with a religious radical who had in her homeland preached against British colonial policy?—or whether the Americans simply changed their minds at the last moment, Ann Lee was delivered only as far as Poughkeepsie, where she, along with Mary Partington, was put into the city jail.

With all the furor over the imprisonment of the Shakers, the commission began releasing the group in October. By November all but Ann Lee and her companion at Poughkeepsie were freed. The group might have spent the entire war behind bars had it not been for the publication of an eyewitness account of Shaker activities written by Valentine Rathbun, an esteemed Massachusetts citizen, who had founded a church in Pittsfield and had, as a member of the state assembly, helped draft Massachusetts's constitution.

Ironically, Rathbun's article constituted a strong attack on the Shakers. He testified that he had once thought of converting to the faith but was now redeemed. He pictured the Shakers as wild and unruly, twitching and squirming during their rites as if possessed by devils and speaking the language of Indians, thus planting suspicion in the minds of many that the Shakers were indeed linked with the British allies, the Iroquois. He called the Shakers "Europeans," and brought up the now-confirmed charge that when men converted to Shakerism, "they . . . immediately throw down their arms, and

cry against the means of defense made use against the common
enemy."

The pacifism of the Shakers was already known to the commissioners and the populace, but the new attack on their ideas
undoubtedly hurt the Shakers. Rathbun went even further, and in a
series of outlandish charges that would eventually mean freedom
for the Shakers, accused them of patently ridiculous crimes. He
wrote:

> The offspring of this scheme is such, that men and their wives have
> parted, children run away from their parents, and society broke up in
> neighborhoods; it makes children deny and disown their parents, and
> say they are full of devils.

The commissioners, upon reading the widely-circulated pamphlet, couldn't align their own perception of the Shakers as a
possibly treasonous group with these new charges of their social and
moral corruption. Rathbun had told of women in the group who ran
through the woods naked, of men who had tried to kill their wives,
of suicides, and of the time when "they hung a woman by the neck,
but took her down before she was dead, to show as a sign how they
were to be persecuted." The Shakers that the commissioners had
seen were quiet, adamant only about their pacifism. They were a
small group; certainly, there was no evidence of their receiving and
corrupting small children or murdering each other.

Rathbun's pamphlet worked to soften the judges toward the
Shakers. Witnessing such obvious distortions about Shaker believers, they began to question whether their own judgments against
them were fair. In October they released Darrow and in November
freed Ann's brother William and John Hocknell. In a few days, all
but Ann and Mary Partington were released, with bonds posted for
all to assure their good behavior.

Rathbun's pamphlet was to cause great difficulties for the Shakers
in their first visits to New England as missionaries, but for now, the
Shaker leaders were free to get Ann Lee out of the jail at Poughkeepsie. William Lee immediately petitioned for his sister's release,
applying to the military commander at Albany, Lieutenant General
James Clinton.

Clinton hesitated to release the leader of the group. He sought
the advice of his brother George Clinton, the governor of the state,
who set up an interview between himself and Shaker leader James

Whittaker. A civil authority such as George Clinton was inclined to be less suspicious than the military one, and the governor became convinced that the Shakers were not attempting to "alienate the minds of the people from their Allegiance to the State." He allowed Ann Lee to post for 200 pounds like the others, "for her good behavior and not saying or consenting to any Matters or Things inconsistent with the Peace and Safety of this the United States." Early in December she was freed with Mary—they were out of jail for the first time in four months.

During her imprisonment the Shakers had become very well known throughout the region, awakening not only fear and curiosity but sympathy as well. During the six months following her release, they received word of dozens of possible converts, many of them upstanding citizens from towns at the New York-Massachusetts border. Word of the Shakers, however, was spreading even farther east into central Massachusetts towns like Harvard and Shirley. By May 1781, the leaders were convinced that a missionary tour would reap substantial numbers of converts.

Ann Lee set off for New England late in May 1781 accompanied by her brother, James Whittaker, and three American converts. The group was heading into a region tormented by great religious divisiveness, and at a time—only four months before the decisive turnabout of American military fortunes at Yorktown, Virginia—when the war was going badly for the Americans. The War of Independence had never received great popular support, and New England was indeed at a great distance from lower New York and the South where the war was now concentrated. But those who feared and opposed Shaker ideas used the issue of their British background to make the overland crusade an oftentimes hellish venture.

At first the mission went smoothly. The group stayed for ten days at Mt. Washington, a small town in extreme western Massachusetts, successfully gaining believers in the isolated area. However, when they turned south toward Connecticut and headed for the Enfield home of David Meacham, brother of Joseph Meacham, they encountered their first hostility. People harassed them with charges of witchcraft; a mob seemed ready to gather up the Shakers and run them out of town, but they took the advice of the town selectmen and left first.

Ann Lee took the band north, stopping at several towns before reaching Harvard, Massachusetts, where she established what was to become a permanent Shaker church. It was a well-chosen site, being the home of the amazingly successful "New Light" preacher Shadrack Ireland. Like Ann Lee he had proclaimed himself a new messiah and had built a house eminently suited for religious radicals who might, quite suddenly, find themselves facing hostile citizens—the house had a secret staircase leading from its roof to its cellar. Ireland, who had died several years before Ann Lee's arrival, had left the area ripe for religious conversions, for he had claimed he would rise three days after his death. His adherents were disillusioned by the failure and awaited yet another savior.

Ann Lee seemed to be just such a messiah. She won the following of several influential men of the town, and soon the entire region was awake to the news of the Shaker activities. Making Harvard her center, Ann Lee journeyed out in all directions for the next year and established Shaker communities not only in nearby towns like Shirley, Hancock, and Enfield, but as far north as New Hampshire and Maine.

The spread of the faith was not accomplished without costs. The potential violence experienced at Enfield was to break out openly several times. Behind the hostilities was the propaganda of Valentine Rathbun, who had written the anti-Shaker tract that had worked to free Ann Lee and other Shakers from their New York jails. Whereas Rathbun seemed outrageous to the commissioners, he was believed by many of the common folk of New England, especially by those who, like himself, saw the Shaker sect as a threat to their own religious groups.

Rathbun continued to exploit the British origins of the Shakers in a number of pamphlets read widely throughout the decade. Rumors about the Shakers became rife. In the summer of 1781, one story circulated throughout Harvard that the Shakers had a cache of wagons and firearms at Shadrack Ireland's house. The captain of the militia searched the house, and even though he found no supplies, he ordered the group out of town.

The Shakers returned to Harvard for short stays throughout the following year, but finally in August 1782 the inevitable outburst occurred. A mob of several hundred people had gathered near the Ireland house, capturing a large Shaker gathering inside. The crowd especially wished to torment Ann Lee but found that she was at Woburn. They attacked the house anyway, bursting through the barred doors and dragging each praying Shaker man and woman from the house one by one. The believers were ordered to leave the town, and when they refused—remaining on their knees in prayer outside the house—the Shaker group was placed between two groups of mounted citizenry and marched from Harvard. They were prodded and whipped, and at one point James Shepherd, the only English Shaker in the group, was beaten with sticks. The mob committed "every kind of abuse that they could invent without taking lives," Shaker testimony reported later.

The influence of the Rathbun pamphlet on the mob action was great. It was an Englishman, not one of the Americans, who was singled out for a severe beating. The group was marched all the way to Lancaster, about ten miles from Harvard, and ordered never to return to the town again. When some of the Shakers did, indeed, proceed immediately to return to Harvard, they were lashed and whipped along the road. One of the Shakers was tied to a tree and his naked body was whipped by men who, echoing a charge by Rathbun, accused the believer of breaking up families.

Ann Lee had luckily avoided the outburst, for she most certainly would have been severely abused had the mob captured her. Her campaign into New England was not to conclude, however, before she faced personal jeopardy. She had escaped being beaten the year before at Petersham when a captain of the local militia turned her over to the Shakers after a "Blackguard Committee" had wrested her in the middle of the night from a Shaker home. A similar outrage marked the end of her New England crusade.

That last trial was to occur in New Lebanon, the town from which the Shakers had received so much early support. They were gathering there in late August 1783, for a number of meetings in farmhouses in the area. Ann Lee had been in New Lebanon for several days before agitation occurred. Unfriendly townspeople began to trace her visits to farms in the area, harassing the leader and her group by calling names at them and knocking loudly at the doors of houses where the group was meeting.

Finally a mob formed before the Shakers could leave the area, as they had planned. While sleeping overnight at the farm of George Darrow, the Shakers were surrounded. In the morning Darrow and David Meacham were seized on the charge that they had abused Meacham's young daughter. The arrest was only a pretense, however, for getting Darrow and Meacham out of the house. The two men were influential in the area, and many in the mob were reluctant to storm Darrow's home while the owner was in it.

While Darrow and Meacham were being taken away for trial, word spread quickly about the threat of violence at the Darrow residence. Soon other Shakers living in the area gathered at the house, gaining entry only after working their way through the hostile mob. David Darrow attempted to convince the mob of their unlawful behavior, and when that failed, the conflict erupted.

The mob charged the house from all sides, breaking through barred doors and dragging out the Shakers by the feet and hair. Those who were difficult to drag were picked up bodily by several men and pitched out the front door. Ann Lee had secreted herself behind a sealed partition at the back of the house, but her hiding place was soon discovered. Breaking through to her sanctuary from an upstairs room by tearing apart the ceiling above her, men dragged the woman to her carriage and ordered one of the Shakers to drive her from the town.

The carriage was driven by Eliab Harlow, a local Shaker farmer. When he had proceeded only about fifteen yards, someone in the unruly crowd managed to cut the reins of the bridle. Harlow attempted to urge the horses on, but several men beat at him and took over the driving of the carriage themselves, planning now to take Ann Lee to the local magistrate.

The ride was perilous. At one point some of the men surrounding the carriage attempted to overturn it when it was crossing over a small bridge. Some of the Shaker men who were accompanying the carriage managed to prevent that disaster, and in the struggle, Thomas Law, one of the leaders of the mob, was injured by falling from his horse. Infuriated, he later pulled one of the elders, James Whittaker, from his horse during the ride to the magistrate's, causing the Shaker leader to fracture three of his ribs.

At the court of the magistrate, Ann Lee—her cap and apron now torn off—was dragged before Eleazar Grant, who was still prosecuting Darrow and Meacham. When he was ready to deal with her, the woman was furious and chastised the magistrate for allowing such lawless activities. "It is your day now," she reproved him loudly, "but it will be mine, by and by; Eleazar Grant, I'll put you into a cockleshell yet."

Grant was in a difficult position, for in the middle of the woman's verbal assault Whittaker attempted to enter a complaint against Law, charging the man with assault. The courthouse was filled with Shakers and their enemies; but present, too, were constables, some of whom did not share a hatred of the religious group. Grant ordered that the proceedings be delayed and Ann Lee was taken away to his house nearby. Later in the day she was brought back with other Shaker leaders and charged with a breach of the peace. Specifically, Grant accused them of making late-night disturbances which woke people from their sleep.

The Shakers denied the charges, and Grant bound them over to County Court. He said they would have to go to jail, but, by law, had to make appeal for bondsmen. The Darrow brothers immediately offered themselves, paid the appropriate bond and led their leaders from the court. Outside, however, a large crowd remained. Grant refused to break them up, and when it was apparent he would not have the constables protect the group, some of the men seized the woman again. They placed her in a carriage, this time bound for Albany.

They took her seven miles over a crude road, followed again by faithful Shakers. They got as far as a tavern on the Albany town line where they stopped for some drinking. The owner of the tavern was shocked at the abuse the woman was receiving; he listened to Shakers who begged for help and decided to assist. He reprimanded the men, threatening to call out constables if the woman was not freed. The group of agitators was dwindling, and they decided they would rather drink than continue the long day's harassment. The Shakers spent the night exhausted in the barn of a nearby farmer, now convinced they would soon have to return to Niskeyuna or face more unspeakable outrages against them.

When they arose in the morning, still weary, wet, and muddy, Ann Lee showed them the bruises on her arms and stomach. Women in the group told the men that she was bruised over her whole body. She told the group she was, finally, getting too tired from the campaign. "I have been like a dying creature," she said, but she resolved to see several more farmers on her return to Niskeyuna. The journey back was marked by more harassment and threats, but in early September the group arrived safely at their New York home.

The long campaign for converts had led to the establishment of several churches in the area, each growing up during the following years around the homes of the faithful in towns like New Lebanon and Harvard. But the crusade seemed as much of a war as the military affair for independence during which it was conducted. Charges that Ann Lee and her English compatriots were British emissaries still continued, and hostility was still enacted against new converts even when the War of Independence ended. Like the larger war, the Shaker campaign had been costly. Ann Lee returned to Niskeyuna wracked by injuries and sickened by her ordeal. Nearly a year after her return, her brother William died. Shortly thereafter on September 8, 1784, convinced that her brother was calling her "to go home," she died. She already was "at home." The Shaker family she had founded in America buried her at Niskeyuna.

13

Mary Katherine Goddard

THE COURAGE to publish the first signed copies of the Declaration of Independence was hers. The ingenuity and determination to maintain regular newspaper publication during the Revolution were hers. But what was not hers, and what ruined the last years of her life, was the legal ownership of her newspaper. Mary Katherine Goddard, America's first woman printer and first woman postmaster, was removed from both these positions in the mid-1780s not because of lack of ability, but because she *was* a talented and successful woman, and therefore, threatening to her male peers.

A person inspired by the Calvinist ethic of duty, work, and renunciation, Mary Katherine's remarkable journalistic and administerial achievements were rewarded not only by her dismissal from the two positions but by familial rejection as well. Her ouster as editor of the *Baltimore Journal*, certainly painful enough in itself, was exacerbated by the fact that her own brother William was himself the perpetrator of her sudden and unwarranted removal.

Mary Katherine, born in June 1738, and her brother William, who was two years younger, were a study in contrasts even during their childhood years in New London, Connecticut, where their father Giles Goddard practiced medicine and ran the local post office. William was born with a hot temper which required a goodly amount of disciplinary action on the part of his mother, since his father was often out making house calls, treating the sick, and managing the post office. Fortunately, she was able to restrain William's temperamental outbursts to a certain extent. The three other Goddard children, of whom only Mary Katherine survived to adulthood, were much less of a problem.

When Giles Goddard died in early 1757, his wife Sarah was

burdened with all the family responsibility. The onslaught of duties connected with heading a family was relieved to some extent for Sarah, since Gile's lucrative endeavors in medicine and mail left his wife an estate worth 780 pounds. At this time Sarah decided to pull up stakes in New London and go to Providence, Rhode Island, to begin a new life. Mary Katherine was nineteen years old at the time of the move, and William was seventeen.

The three remaining Goddards had all developed an interest in the printing business. William, presumably because he was the sole male, was the one who could most readily act on that desire. In 1755 while the Goddards were still residing in New London, William had become apprenticed to James Parker at the *Connecticut Gazette,* established that year with John Holt. Parker and Holt also established in 1760 the *New-York Gazette and Weekly Post-Boy.* William probably worked in both New Haven and New York for Holt and Parker. The apprenticeship lasted until 1762 when William embarked on an independent printing career. William's travels back and forth between New Haven and New York proved to be the model for his entire life. Restlessness and curiosity compelled him to move from one city to another, either to establish new business ventures and newspapers or to escape the repercussions of the political controversy in which the hotheaded William often found himself embroiled.

At the conclusion of his apprenticeship and with 300 pounds support from his mother, William opened a newspaper, thereby becoming the first newspaper publisher in Rhode Island. On August 31, 1762, he published a prospectus for the *Providence Gazette and Country Journal,* the first issue of which appeared in October of that year. This paper contained an article, by William, "To the Publick", in which he spoke of the "utility and advantages" of the printing business. In regard to the Seven Years' War then going on between France, England, and other nations, William stated on page one: "Every Thing that relates to the Honour and Interest of our Country, and the Humiliation of our Enemies, must be peculiarly interesting and as such, they shall be carefully inserted in the Paper." This premier statement of aims and attitudes indicates more than William's editorial policy. The patriotism bordering on fanaticism and the hotheadedness lurking in this statement accompanied William in all his endeavors, political and editorial.

The publication of the *Providence Gazette* required much physical exertion. The standard hand press of the eighteenth century printed approximately 200 papers per hour. Leather balls performed the inking, which required one page to be inked twice so that both sides were printed. By 1763 the *Gazette* was advertising for both an apprentice and a journeyman, since the work was exceeding the capacities of the Goddard trio. The *Gazette,* a three-column folio, required the setting of about 22,000 ems for an issue. At least four days of each week were needed for one printer to do the composition and presswork. It was in these early days of the *Gazette* that Mary Katherine became expert in the technical side of publishing.

The Goddards' other printing ventures at this time included a broadside proclaiming the fall of Moro Castle at Havana, a playbill for a production later banned, and sermons—that ever popular eighteenth-century literary form.

In spite of this auspicious beginning, William was unable to obtain adequate support for the *Gazette,* and therefore decided to leave town. After three years of financial losses and dwindling subscriptions, *Gazette* publication stopped. The management of the remaining printing work was left to Sarah and Mary Katherine. The Goddard women published *West's Almanack* and other publications under the name of "Sarah and William Goddard." By August 1766 Sarah managed to reopen the *Gazette* under the heading of "Sarah Goddard and Company." The "Company" consisted mostly of daughter Mary Katherine. The two women managed the newspaper, a bookstore, and a bookbindery. Among the publications of the press was the first American edition of Lady Mary Wortley Montagu's letters, printed under the title *Letters of the Right Honourable Lady M--y W-----y M------u.*

By 1765, however, the family decided to sell the Providence newspaper to John Carter so that Mary Katherine and Sarah could join William in Philadelphia, where he had established the *Pennsylvania Chronicle and Universal Advertiser.* William's printing interests in Philadelphia had begun with Joseph Galloway and Thomas Wharton, when the three had set up a printing business. Internal conflict, however, soon led to the dissolving of the partnership. Much of the financial responsibility for the *Chronicle* was assumed by Sarah, and, as usual, William depended heavily on the assistance of both Sarah and Mary Katherine in getting out the newspaper.

This arrangement abruptly ended in January 1770 when Sarah died at the age of seventy, thereby removing the last effective control over William's erratic ways. Since William was in New York at the time, Mary Katherine was confronted alone not only with the grief arising from the death of her mother but also with vulture-businessmen who, playing on her shocked state and what they viewed as her womanly naivete, bared their talons in order to attack what they considered an easy prey. One of these men, Joseph Galloway, pressured her to sell the *Pennsylvania Chronicle* for a small sum by arguing that William would remain in New York. Mary Katherine stood firmly against this profiteering, however, and informed Galloway that she had no intention whatsoever of selling the business. William later wrote of the affair:

> On the death of my mother, he [Galloway] paid my sister a visit; and after condoling with her for the great loss she had sustained, for which he expressed the utmost concern, . . . he pulled a paper from his pocket, containing an estimate of the value of my business, and by a *false view* of it, endeavored to prevail on my sister to sell it for a trifle; for says he, 'your brother will not, he cannot return here—you have no friends here—you would live much happier in *New England*—and may make something for yourself by a sale of this interest.' My sister saw his baseness, and that he was a man who could smile with a dagger in his hand, told him that she knew the business was very valuable, and that she should listen to no such proposals. To this she generously added, that although by the sudden death of my mother, one half of the interest became hers, by law, yet she would give it all up to me, as it was designed for me.

William's view of the affair reveals not only the brotherly concern and indignation he took pains to display, but the connivance he used in obtaining ownership of the *Pennsylvania Chronicle*. William made the self-righteous assumption that his mother meant him to inherit full ownership of the operation. Of course men in the eighteenth century, as in the twentieth, did own most of the property. But whether Sarah intended to leave William all of her most valuable property seems highly questionable. The fact that Sarah Goddard was herself a successful publisher and business-woman leads one to believe that she would want a career for her daughter Mary Katherine, whose decision not to marry necessitated her self-support. William was, of course, free to speculate blatantly about the wishes of his now-dead mother, since she was not available to affirm or deny his contentions. However, it remains highly suspect that Sarah Goddard would harken only to the wishes of her son and ignore the best interests of her daughter.

Whether Mary Katherine ever hoped or intended to marry will

remain unknown, since all of her letters and private papers have been lost. It seems likely that, even had she married and received her livelihood from her husband, she would have wanted to continue her newspaper work. The example Sarah had already set of running a household and assisting on the newspaper would have deeply impressed her daughter and could have led her to want the same kind of varied life.

Having successfully resisted opportunists like Galloway, Mary Katherine was left in Philadelphia to run the *Pennsylvania Chronicle*, just as she and her mother had been left before to cope with the floundering *Providence Gazette*. William was spending most of his time in Baltimore in 1773 and 1774 establishing the *Baltimore Journal*. The last issue of the *Chronicle* appeared February 8, 1774. Nine days later Mary Katherine began running the *Journal*, the press which William had purchased from Nicholas Hasselbach, Baltimore's first printer.

In his usual pattern, William then left Baltimore to establish not another newspaper but this time the intercolonial postal system. This departure from newspaper publishing did not dim William's intense interest in the concept of freedom of the press.

Both William and Mary Katherine were active in their concern for press freedom in America. Mary Katherine's more relaxed temperament prevented her from engaging in the sometimes violent political fighting that William seemed to relish. But in her own more levelheaded way Mary Katherine defended the values of liberty. At one point, she was verbally abused by George Somerville, a Baltimore citizen who was angered by some of Mary Katherine's published remarks about him. Unwilling to take such threats lightly, she reported the man to the proper authorities—in this case the County Committee. The records of the committee's proceedings indicate that Mary Katherine was, indeed, justified in her action:

> Miss Goddard informed this Committee, by Letter, that on Wednesday last Mr. George Somerville came to her office and abused her with threats and indecent language on account of a late publication in her paper. The Committee, conceiving it to be their duty to inquire into everything that has a tendency to restrain the liberty of the Press, *Ordered*, that a summons be issued for the said George Somerville, returnable at three o'clock p.m.

After refusing the summons, Somerville was brought directly before the committee, censured, and released on bond.

This toughness of mind and dogged determination enabled Mary Katherine to maintain regular publication of the *Baltimore Journal* during the trying years of the Revolution, when runaway inflation and lack of paper made publication of any kind a difficult task. While many colonial newspapers were forced to capitulate to these wartime conditions, Mary Katherine refused to do so. The primary reason she was able to continue regular publication was due to her obtaining sufficient supplies of newsprint from a paper mill established by William with Eleazer Oswald in April 1777. Having overcome the paper problem, Mary Katherine coped with the inflation by raising subscription rates. Her dramatic increases indicated the severity of the inflation that harassed the colonists. The yearly rate of ten shillings charged in 1773, was doubled by 1777. A year later, it had more than doubled again, going to fifty-two shillings, and by 1779 the rate had skyrocketed to ten pounds annually.

Having met and overcome these immense problems, Mary Katherine valiantly forged ahead in her endeavor to provide her contemporaries with accurate news and incisive reporting. These qualities of accuracy and thorough reportage led to the journalistic coup of her career. In January 1777 she published the first copy of the Declaration of Independence that contained all the names of the signers. Other newspapers had published the Declaration earlier but none of them carried the names of the signers. This kind of first-rate reporting, coupled with the Goddards' paper source, enabled the *Baltimore Journal* to hold one of the best publication records of any wartime newspaper.

Mary Katherine had also been involved in bookbinding in her printing shop that was associated with the *Baltimore Journal.* In the February 2, 1779 edition of the *Journal,* she advertised many books sold "cheap, for cash." About the same time, Mary Katherine's chief newspaper competitor, the *Maryland Gazette,* was forced to close due primarily to a shortage of paper. Beginning what was to become an American tradition, the Goddards had forced out the competition by helping to make paper unavailable to them.

Although Mary Katherine and her publishing were essentially left alone by William during the war years, he made his presence felt on a few occasions. One serious instance of William's encroaching on what had become Mary Katherine's operation occurred in May 1781. Along with the bookbinding, bookselling, and newspaper publication associated with the *Journal,* Mary Katherine had established a successful system of almanac publication and distribution, taking advantage of the motley uses to which almanacs were put at the time. By 1779 Mary Katherine was printing her own almanacs and those published in German by Matthias Bartgis in Fredericks-town, Maryland. William came to Baltimore while he was working on the postal system, saw the huge success his sister had made of the *Journal* and its offshoots, and decided he must conquer. Mary Katherine, although devoted to her brother, was not anxious for him to win control over the businesses she had so assiduously and painstakingly set up. Her main consideration was not so much selfishness as it was a realization of her brother's penchant for involving himself in bitter and dangerous controversies. For years Mary Katherine and others had stood on the sidelines and watched William engage himself in violently controversial and dangerous activities.

One instance of Mary Katherine's unflagging devotion to her unpredictable brother occurred in late 1776 when William delivered for publication two articles, one of which, signed "Tom Tell-Truth," satirically advocated American acquiescence to British wishes. The second article, signed "Caveto," urged renewed effort by Americans to resist British demands. Both articles were intended to point out to Americans their failure to stand firm against the oppressive mother country. When the Whig Club, an organization so fervently patriotic it approached blindness on some issues, misread the first article as a serious proposal to capitulate to the British, they were provoked to immediate action. They chose to ignore the "Caveto" article, with which they agreed, focusing instead on the identity of "Tom Tell-Truth."

An irony even more pronounced than that intended in the "Tom" article occurred when the illustrious representatives of the Whig Club approached Samuel Chase, eminent Maryland signer of the Declaration of Independence, for advice as to what action should be taken against Mary Katherine for printing such an outrage. Little did the Whig Clubbers know that Chase himself was Tom Tell-Truth and Caveto. Unable to take the club representatives serious-ly, Chase responded, "Why don't you tar and feather her?" His levity indicated that Chase and the Goddards assumed that their *Journal* readership was too sophisticated to take the irony literally.

But what had begun as a caution in the guise of humor ended in a life-and-death confrontation involving violence, exile, and finally, state intervention. The Whig Club first approached Mary Katherine in order to determine the identity of the author of the article. She refused to identify the author and referred the club representatives to William, who had delivered the articles to the *Journal.* In marked contrast to his sister's subdued response, William answered the club's demands by roaring forth with wild polemics about freedom of the press and the right to protection. No evidence indicates that William attempted to explain the ironic nature of the articles to the club and thereby to conciliate them. He seemed to relish the confrontation, and the club reacted by carrying him bodily to their meeting at Rusk's Tavern for questioning. The club ordered William to leave town within the next twenty-four hours. He immediately set off for Annapolis, not in compliance with the club's demands, but to seek help from the government of Maryland, which he obtained. Returning to Baltimore, William proceeded to print *The Prowess of the Whig Club,* a stinging denouncement of the group that provoked the club to vote again for the exile of this "dangerous Tory sympathizer." The nature of William's *Prowess* pamphlet is aptly indicated in the quotation from Jonathan Swift which appeared on the title page: "These Demoniacs let me dub/With the Name of LEGION-CLUB." Before William was able once more to receive help from the state, the Whig Club radicals marched to the Goddard press, again seized the resisting hothead, and conveyed him to Rusk's Tavern for questioning.

Immediately after his seizure, Mary Katherine set out to obtain police help for her brother. Her many visits to Baltimore officials proved fruitless, however, as the city's legal system lay in disarray from the effects of the war. The affair died down after Governor Thomas Johnson ordered the Whig Club to cease and desist its gang activities against William. On his return to Baltimore, he planned further publications railing against the bandit-like tactics of the club. In this case, though, Mary Katherine toned down the vituperative nature of the publications, thereby helping to assure that further violence would be avoided.

The Whig Club's confrontations illustrate only one of the many volatile situations in which William continually placed himself. In each case Mary Katherine had come to his aid. Little wonder, then, that Mary Katherine was reluctant to transfer her power at the *Journal* and printing shop to William, the ever wild one, and to sacrifice what she considered to be her own printing establishment. It was probably evident to her that any transfer of power to her brother would likely involve more battles between William and his numerous enemies. The very survival of the newspaper was at stake. Indeed, the survival of Mary Katherine herself must have been an important consideration for her, since she derived much of her livelihood from the *Journal*, as well as much of her happiness.

However, William insisted and managed to overcome his sister's protests. On January 2, 1784, it was announced that the *Baltimore Journal* would be published by William and Mary Katherine Goddard. In the next issue on January 6, Mary Katherine's name did not appear in the newspaper, and her name never again graced the *Baltimore Journal.*

The most prominent evidence of the beginning of the split between brother and sister was the publication by each, separately, of the annual almanac in 1784. Mary Katherine had been regularly printing the *Pennsylvania, Delaware, Maryland, and Virginia Almanack* since 1780. In 1784, however, there appeared two Goddard almanacs—*Mary Katherine Goddard's Pennsylvania, Delaware, Maryland, and Virginia Almanack* and *William Goddard's Pennsylvania, Delaware, Maryland, and Virginia Almanack.* Probably the decisive factor in this sibling showdown was William's blatant public attack on his only sister—similar to so many of his previous verbal assaults on various and sundry people—and on his sister's almanac:

> Observing a spurious Performance, containing a mean, vulgar, and common-place Selection of Articles . . . I find myself obliged to inform the Public, that the above-mentioned *spurious double-faced Almanack*, is only a *Pennsylvania* one, under a *Baltimore* Mask, of Title-Page, and which was printed in *Philadelphia*, and sent to the *Market* by a certain *hypocritical Character*, for the dirty and mean Purpose of Fraud and Deception.

Certainly private family feuds are painful and difficult enough. But to air publicly the family linen via one's newspaper is even more trying. In her quiet dignified way, Mary Katherine did not respond to her brother's disgusting accusation via the newspaper. She did, however, institute five lawsuits against him, all of which she soon dropped. Their relationship remained severed for the rest of their lives. On numerous occasions mutual friends attempted to bring about a reconciliation, but their efforts were fruitless.

The harsh treatment accorded Mary Katherine by her brother appears in an even darker light when one discovers that William eventually sold the *Baltimore Journal.* On January 11, 1785, it was revealed that Edward Langworthy would become a new partner in the business. Langworthy left the operation eventually; William's brother-in-law, James Agnell, became a new partner in August 1789 and bought the paper in 1792. Again, one concludes that William was simply unable to remain at one job for an extended period of time.

It is likely that William's inflammatory temperament and ability to hold grudges for remarkable lengths of time prevented him from allowing his sister to share the newspaper operation after their 1784 quarrel. Although severely disappointed about her loss of control of her successful operation, Mary Katherine initially was able to take solace from her years of work in another area. She had been appointed postmistress of Baltimore in the fall of 1775, thereby becoming the first woman ever to assume that position in America. Her ability to manage a post office had been acquired from her father, who had successfully managed the New London post office for many years.

Because of William's pioneering work in the colonial postal system, designed to supplant the British system, he is considered the father of the U.S. Postal System. The work he did in that field was the result of one of his jaunts away from his publishing interests and was one of the many times that William left the printing responsibility on Mary Katherine's shoulders.

Much of the basis for William's success in establishing the colonial postal system was the American resentment toward the British postal service. William provided a viable alternative to that system, creating the embryo of what would become an extensive and effective network for written communication in the United States. William worked long and hard in his endeavor to set up the postal system and achieved undeniable success in putting together a workable network of post offices and effective transportation between them. Because of his diligence and success in the establishment of the colonial postal alternative to the British, William expected to be rewarded for his efforts by receiving the second highest post when Congress took over the system. Benjamin Franklin was placed in the top slot. William was defeated by nepotism, however, and Franklin's son-in-law, Richard Bache, was awarded the second post. William was offered a choice between the much less important positions of postmaster of Baltimore or the surveyorship of the system. William chose the surveyorship, while Mary

Katherine was given the job of postmistress of Baltimore, another appointment bearing traces of nepotism.

Mary Katherine undertook her postal duties with the self-discipline and sense of duty that had characterized her work in journalism and business. Under her leadership, the Baltimore post office ran smoothly and efficiently, in spite of the fact that she was devoting much of her energy to the *Baltimore Journal.* In 1784 she established a delivery service, further enhancing the local postal operation. But innovative ideas, hard work, and determination were unable to prevent Mary Katherine from being summarily dismissed from the post office, just as those qualities had been unable to redeem her in her loss of the *Journal.* The fact that Mary Katherine had, during her fourteen years as postmistress, kept the Baltimore post office in operation by using her personal funds was, along with her other contributions, ignored by her superiors in the postal system.

In 1789 Mary Katherine was instantly removed from her position as postmistress of Baltimore. Clearly the victim of a power play by political superiors, she was informed that her dismissal was due to the fact that as a woman she would be unable to maintain the long-distance riding on horseback that the position would require when Baltimore became a regional center. The fact that this "explanation" was completely phony is evidenced by the utter absence of any such horseback commuting by the newly appointed Baltimore postmaster, John White.

Mary Katherine fell into a state of shock. First her brother William, the object of so much sisterly pride and protection, had shunned and publicly denounced her, resulting in her loss of the *Baltimore Journal* she had grown to love. Now seemingly anonymous men removed her from her other career as postmistress of a growing city. While the Revolution raged on American soil and times were difficult for everyone, Mary Katherine's services were called for and she responded immediately and selflessly. With the cessation of hostilities, with the opening of new opportunities for the new citizens of the United States of America, Mary Katherine was thrust aside, forgotten by those whom she had aided so effectively in times of need.

Unlike her first summary dismissal, Mary Katherine did not blithely acquiesce to her firing from the postal system. She immediately enlisted the help of her many friends and associates in the Baltimore business community, who readily exerted all the power at their command to reinstate her as postmistress of Baltimore. Samuel Osgood, the postmaster general, was approached with a petition dated November 12, 1789, requesting Mary Katherine's reinstatement. More than 230 signatures of prominent Maryland citizens appeared on the petition, including those of the governor of Maryland and the French consul. After delaying for some time, Osgood refused to meet the request of the petition. Mary Katherine's next step was an appeal to President George Washington. He managed to sidestep the issue by saying that he wished not to interfere in the internal affairs of the postal department. The United States Senate was the next object of Mary Katherine's appeal. On January 29, 1790, she appealed to the Senate, but as in her previous attempts, futility prevailed.

More salt was poured on Mary Katherine's psychic wounds when White died soon after his appointment, and she was refused the post again, in spite of the fact that she was the logical choice as White's successor. Fourteen years of hard work in the Baltimore post office were rewarded by silence and intentional apathy on the part of her superiors.

Although Mary Katherine had had her newspaper and her post office brutally taken from her, she managed to maintain the small dry goods establishment and bookstore she had set up in the early years of the Revolution. These business ventures sustained Mary Katherine in the last, somewhat embittered years of her life. On August 12, 1816, she died at the age of eighty. In her will she freed her devoted black servant, Belinda Starling, and left her all her property. William was not mentioned in the will.

14

Patience Wright

PATIENCE WRIGHT was the first American to achieve success in sculpture. Her success is all the more remarkable for her lack of formal training in art or any formal education at all. She had a great talent which she developed herself without commercial motives. It was later in life when, as a widow with five children to support, she developed her art into a successful business.

Patience was born in 1725 in Bordentown, New Jersey, as Patience Lovell. The Lovell family had originally been established at Oyster Bay, Long Island. It was a large and closely knit clan that had expanded from Oyster Bay to New Jersey and to Newport, Rhode Island, where Patience's cousin Robert Feke—who painted the first portrait of Benjamin Franklin—had settled.

Her mother was Patience Townsend, and her father, John Lovell, was a prosperous farmer who was well liked by the other residents of Bordentown. His Quaker faith provided the base for his education of the children, who were not formally schooled but raised with directness and simplicity of manner. The family was large; there were ten children, though we know only of seven—Patience, her sister Rachel, a brother John, and four other sisters.

By Patience's own accounts, the family lived well on a large farm populated with all kinds of domestic animals. The children were trained in the arts of farming, dairying, and housekeeping. Lovell was convinced that it was counter to the Lord's will to kill His animal creatures to feed His human creatures, and so he imposed a strict vegetarian diet on the family. In addition, he insisted that the entire family dress in white from head to foot. The Lovells must have been not only popular but also highly visible.

This strict regulation of their lives did not prevent the children from developing their own personalities, and Patience claimed that the strict discipline of the home was what moved her and her sister Rachel to begin modeling figures as children. They used clay and soft bread to mold the figures, and from herbs, flowers, and the sap of trees, they made dyes for coloring them.

Such interests were not customary in Quaker life, but John Lovell apparently did nothing to stop Patience. If he had, it would have done no good, for Patience was a headstrong young woman.

Patience's parents could not have known at her baptism how ironic was the name they gave her, for she was anything but patient. In her early twenties, she ran off to Philadelphia hoping to find success in the big city. She was encouraged to do so by Francis Hopkinson, a painter who lived across the road from the Lovells and who probably led her to use wax for her models. Patience saw that in a city like Philadelphia she would have an opportunity to make a successful career for herself as a wax modeler.

By this time waxwork shows had been a popular entertainment in Europe and the colonies for some time. The figures were usually not well modeled, and normally they were either of beings that had never existed or of people already dead. Mythological, religious, criminal, royal, humorous, and horrific figures were the popular types.

Patience was already a skillful modeler when she went to Philadelphia, but if she intended to make it as a commercial artist there, her plans were quickly short-circuited, for she married in 1748 at the age of twenty-three. Her husband was Joseph Wright, a cooper much older than she. Patience married him at the urging of her father, who was probably a friend of Wright's; the latter, like Lovell, was from Bordentown and his family, too, was originally from Oyster Bay. Lovell must have found in Wright someone who would settle down the rambunctious and restless Patience.

Her marriage to Wright lasted until his death in 1769. She was then immediately faced with the problem of supporting their five children.

Patience began working in wax models again, and with her sister Rachel, who was also a wax modeler, she established a show that toured the cities of the American coast. It was very successful; crowds came from everywhere to the exhibits. Newspapers praised the show, and Patience came to know many people, including the Franklin family in Philadelphia and Jane Mecom, Franklin's sister in Boston.

Patience is a landmark figure in wax modeling, for she started in America the kind of wax museums we have now. Her figures were of famous people still alive, and often of major figures in the center of America's struggle to become an independent country. One of her busts, for example, was of Benjamin Franklin. Fifty years before the invention of photography, her wax displays presented the great figures of political and cultural life to the people.

Patience was an extremely skillful modeler; her figures were lifelike in their detail and coloring. They were made with hollow, light heads and bodies and dressed with real clothing. A figure she made of Franklin was even dressed in a suit of Franklin's own clothing which he had given to her for the purpose.

Because of the poor heating systems of the time, summer was the best season for modeling figures—the wax was softer and more pliable. Patience put the head in her lap under her apron for warmth and molded its features with her fingers while keeping her eyes on the face of the sitter, whose attention she held with a constant babbling monologue.

Wax is not a very rugged material, however, and only one of the figures Patience made is left to us today; even this is in damaged condition. It is of the pro-American English politician William Pitt, Lord Chatham, and is kept in Westminster Abbey. However, from the testimony of those who knew Patience or saw her works, we have other evidence of the incredible fidelity to life of her figures and of the delight people took in them.

New York was more or less Patience's home in these years of travel. While she and Rachel were partners in the wax show, Patience was the owner and Rachel received a twenty-five percent share of the profits. Elizabeth Wright, Patience's eldest daughter, worked as manager of the show. Another daughter, Phoebe, was also with her in New York and her only son, Joseph—who was later to become a portrait painter—was in school in Philadelphia. Patience was well known in New York, and three prominent men of the city were advisors to her family.

New York was also the scene of a disaster for Patience. On June 3, 1771, she and Rachel were out of the house when one of the children started a fire in the waxworks. The blaze spread and engulfed the house. Before it was put out, it had nearly destroyed the house and had ruined almost all of the figures.

The show, of course, had to be closed, but Patience immediately set to work rebuilding it. She added new figures and replaced the lost ones, and just two months later she opened the show again with great success.

The popularity of her figures led her to move to England. She felt confident that she could produce a wax show that would appeal to a large public, and she knew that in England there was a larger audience than in America, with its smaller population and fewer cities. With the same desire for the opportunities offered by larger and more cosmopolitan places that had led her to leave Bordentown for Philadelphia, at the age of forty-seven Patience decided to leave America to find greater success in London.

She packed up her wax figures, left the children to be sent for later, and sailed for England in February 1772 on the ship *Nancy*. She arrived in London in late March, and she arrived prepared. She not only had letters of introduction from important Americans, but also a letter from Jane Mecom asking Franklin to help her get established. She brought with her a wax bust of Cadwaller Colden, the lieutenant governor of New York and a close friend of Franklin's; he was delighted with her sculpture of his friend.

Franklin did his best to aid Patience. He was in London to build sympathy for the American cause among English politicians and other influential people, and he had a large circle of friends. Through Franklin, Patience met David Garrick, the actor; Catherine Macaulay, the liberal historian; and most importantly, William Pitt, Lord Chatham, who became a friend and correspondent through all her years in London. She made wax models of all these people, and in this way not only complimented them but also created appealing figures for her exhibit.

In London society she found both subjects for her modeling and audiences for her shows. She established a studio and an exhibition room in Pall Mall, London's most fashionable district, and settled down to several years of great success.

The English press gave serious recognition to Patience's artistic skill. The realism of her figures was disturbing, for people would see life-size representations of their friends in perfect detail, except that the figures did not move—their deathly quiet disturbed quite a few individuals.

Some of her visitors provide us with anecdotes about her and her work. One English Lady came into a room and spoke to a housemaid; when the housemaid did not answer, the Lady discovered that she was one of Patience's wax figures. Mrs. John Adams found, in Patience's studio, an old clergyman sitting in a chair

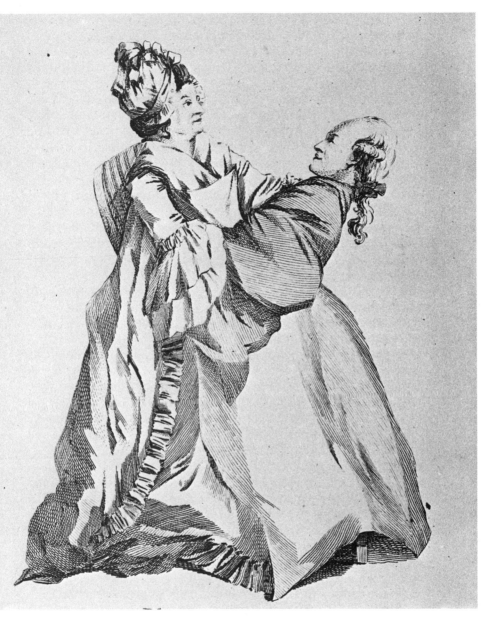

*Patience Wright with one of her figures, said to be Dr. William
Dodd. (Engraving from London Magazine)
Courtesy, Charles Coleman Sellers*

reading a newspaper. She watched him for ten minutes before she realized that he too was made of wax. A friend of Franklin's who had just listened to Franklin advise him to get married, said that instead he would have Mrs. Wright make him a wife to sit at the dinner table with him.

In spite of her success, Patience was not free of political and personal difficulties. A rift grew between her and Franklin. He wrote to his wife Deborah in 1773 that he thought he had offended Patience somehow, for she was avoiding him. She had, moreover, removed from her exhibit a bust which she had made of Franklin when she first came to London.

But all this was not due to any offense. What had happened was that Patience had met Thomas Penn and his wife, Lady Juliana. She made wax models of both, and they became her patrons. Too, they introduced her to the king and queen, whom she endeared with her simplicity and direct manner—she called them not "Your Majesty" but George and Charlotte.

The Penn family and Franklin were bitter enemies for both political and personal reasons, and Patience had removed the figure of Franklin from her show to accommodate them. Into the show went busts of the Penns and of the king and queen.

For their part, the Penns thought that Patience's art could be used as political propaganda. Since the Penns were hated in Pennsylvania, they felt that this hostility would diminish if they could remind the people of their actual selves. Patience made a bust of Thomas Penn which she then sent to the Pennsylvania Assembly with instructions to place it in the public library of Philadelphia and have it cared for by Rachel Wells.

Patience did not completely break off with Franklin; she was simply being diplomatic. Later, after the war had started and Franklin was in Paris getting French assistance for America, Patience wrote advising him of information she had heard from important people who came to her show.

She realized, after her show had been going on for some time, that the politically influential persons who came to it were a mine of information on English plans and policies. She tried to discover things from them in conversation and then wrote to Franklin. She saw herself as an informant in the enemy camp, but actually she said little about the war in her letters, which were filled with praises for Franklin, apologies for bothering him, and much personal news. There was a series of letters in which she asked for his aid in getting her daughter's fiance, an American prisoner of war named Ebenezer Platt, out of jail. A letter from Franklin secured Platt's release. Patience's correspondence with Franklin was on the whole incoherent, disorganized, and difficult to read because of her poor handwriting and complete lack of grammatical knowledge. She certainly did not deserve the reputation she acquired as America's first woman spy. Nonetheless Franklin liked her, though he sometimes found her to be more a humorous figure than anything else.

Patience did not lose contact with America or her friends there, either. During her London years, the wax show in New York was kept going by Rachel, and Patience would send her figures of famous English people she had met. These included the king and queen, William Pitt, John Wesley, and George Whitefield; she also sent Rachel a bust of Franklin.

Patience was an outspoken American sympathizer and activist in London during the war. She announced her views and support of American independence to everyone in English society regardless of their own position on the issue. This cost her the friendship of the king when she directly criticized him for the war while he was visiting her salon. Her house was a refuge for American prisoners of war, and she exchanged information with English politicians who supported the American cause.

She wrote often as well to William Pitt, who developed a dossier on her which he probably gave to Franklin later in Paris.

Her period of political activism began in 1774. She not only began gleaning information from her audiences, but she also tried to aid the American cause through domestic politics. She helped John Sawbridge, the brother of Catherine Macaulay, in his campaign for the parliamentary elections of that autumn. The election that year was based on a grass roots movement to reform government by ousting corrupt officials and liberalizing policy, and Patience hoped that out of this reform, war between England and America could be avoided.

Her daughter Phoebe had married John Hoppner, an English portrait painter. Hoppner had been raised and trained under the auspices of the crown, but upon his marriage to Phoebe he was thrown out penniless. Patience blamed Benjamin West, another painter, for this, but it was not his doing. West did not like Patience, but he had never attempted to injure her fortunes and, in fact, greatly helped her son Joseph when he went to Paris to study painting in 1780, despite a scandal he had caused.

Joseph showed promise as a painter, and in 1780 he exhibited a painting at the Royal Academy. It was a portrait of Patience working on a wax head with the king and queen as onlookers. Patience, in turn, was conversing with the royal couple as she worked. The scandal occurred when the painting was publicly hung and people discovered that the head she was modeling was that of Charles I, the king beheaded after the Revolution of 1648. The painting shockingly implied that King George was next in line for beheading. At this time with the war going badly for the English, serious political conflicts within the country, and talk of revolution and overthrow in the air, such a painting bordered on sedition.

The scandal, however, did not affect Patience's fortunes directly. Her desire to go to Paris was not a wish to escape her London troubles, but was founded on her desire to achieve greater success, like her moves to Philadelphia and London. She hoped to set up a wax exhibit and conquer the French as she had the English.

In March 1779 Patience had written to Franklin, explaining that she had moved from Pall Mall, was settling her affairs, and wanted to return to America after visiting him in Paris. Franklin was not happy to hear this; he wrote back to her that he was looking forward to seeing her, but that she should forget about trying to establish herself in Paris. He presented a list of discouraging problems she would have to face—competition from other wax artists, the waning appeal of wax shows in Paris, and the high cost of living there. In a postscript he claimed was from his grandson (whom Patience had known as a little boy), she was advised that her lifelike figures would require passports, which would be a great expense to her and a contribution to the English treasury as well.

Franklin's ploy didn't work. Patience came to Paris in 1780 in the midst of the scandal provoked by Joseph's painting. Franklin received her graciously, and she did another wax model of him which she eventually dressed in a suit of his own clothes.

A ridiculous incident caused by this model testifies to the realism of Patience's figures. Franklin was living at Passy, a suburb on the Right Bank, and Patience decided to walk over one evening and present the model to him. On the way she was stopped at a roadblock by the police, who were checking travelers for contraband. They insisted she open the bundle she was carrying. Patience was outraged at this invasion of privacy and flatly refused. This only fired the suspicions and determination of the police who took the bundle from her by force and proceeded to open it. They were astounded to find in it the head of a man. It was dark. Patience could not speak French and the police could not speak English. Patience was shouting and raving in her outrage. Without further discussion, the police closed the bundle and arrested Patience. They had decided that she was an escaped lunatic who had murdered a man and was on her way to dispose of the head.

On the way to the police station Patience somehow persuaded the officers to stop at the apartment of a friend, Elkanah Watson. He was finally able to explain it all to the police, and everyone was left laughing at the absurdity of the whole affair except for Patience, who continued raging.

Unfortunately this incident wasn't the only difficulty that Patience faced during her time there. She found that Franklin had been accurate in his estimate of the problems she would have setting up in Paris. The wax show audience there was well covered by Philippe Curtiss, the uncle of Madame Tussaud, and there was no room for another wax artist. When she became convinced of this, Patience decided to return to London.

Patience's inability to establish herself in Paris marked the beginning of a decline in her fortunes. She was fifty-six years old when she returned to London in 1781, and she found that she was no longer as popular in society as she once had been. Her personal vitality remained strong, though, and she still wanted to return to her native country.

She was also still an ardent Patriot and admirer of the men who had led America through the Revolution. In 1783 she wrote to Washington in the United States telling him of her desire to return and do a wax bust of him. Her letter took a full year to reach Washington, and by this time Joseph had visited Washington and done a wax mask and a portrait of him. Washington replied graciously that he would be honored to be counted among the numerous friends who would welcome her back to her native country.

A year later, though, Patience was still in London, and she never did get to do a bust of Washington from life. However, from the painting and the mask that Joseph had done, she was able to model a fine wax medallion of him. She had also intended to do a bust of Jefferson, and in the summer of 1785 she wrote to him in Paris, but again her ambition was not fulfilled. She did not go to Paris again, nor did she return to America. In February 1786 she was returning from a visit with John Adams, the American ambassador to England, when she fell on the street and died soon afterward.

Her sister Rachel survived her and lived out her years as a recluse among wax figures. Joseph died early, as did Elizabeth and Ebenezer Platt.

Patience was a talented and eccentric woman, and her personality, though strong, did not leave a noble impression of our first sculptor.

The best accounts of her character come from two prominent Americans who met her in Europe.

Elkanah Watson met Patience by chance in Paris in 1781. He found her an overwhelming personality—she did not so much relate to people she met as engulf them in her energy. Watson was calling to his servant from the balcony of his room when he suddenly "was assailed by a powerful female voice, crying out from an upper story, 'Who are you? An American, I hope.' 'Yes, Madam,' I replied, 'and who are you?' In two minutes she came blustering downstairs, with the familiarity of an old acquaintance." Watson found that her appearance suited her personality well, for "the wild flights of her powerful mind stamped originality on all her acts and language. She was tall and athletic in figure; walked with a firm, bold step, and erect as an Indian. Her complexion was somewhat sallow—her cheekbones high—her face furrowed, and olive eyes keen, piercing, and expressive. Her sharp glance was appalling; it had almost the wildness of the maniac," and "she would utter language that would put her hearers to the blush." In Watson's case at least, such a stormy meeting began a lasting friendship, and he often was of great aid to Patience and her family in Europe.

If Watson appreciated Patience's eccentricities and rambunctiousness, others were not so responsive to her. Mrs. John Adams was one of these; she met her in London in 1784 and was repelled by her. Patience was as aggressive toward the famous Mrs. Adams as she had been to Watson years earlier. Mrs. Adams wrote that she "caught me by the hand. 'Why, is it really and in truth Mrs. Adams, and is that your daughter? Why you dear soul how young you look. Well I am glad to see you. All of you Americans? Well I must kiss you all.' Having passed the ceremony upon me and Abby she runs to the gentlemen. 'I make no distinction,' says she, and gave them each a hearty kiss from which we all rather have been excused for her appearance is quite the slattern."

Patience held Mrs. Adams with her rambling conversation for half an hour. Mrs. Adams concluded that Patience was "the queen of sluts, and her tongue runs like Unity Bedlam's." Mrs. Adams usually had a low opinion of the women she met in Europe, but her description of Patience's behavior so matches Watson's that we must accept it. The difference is that where Watson appreciated Patience, Mrs. Adams rejected her for her lack of gentility.

The English, however, had found this absence of formality in Patience refreshing. At the time America was known to Europeans in only mythical ways. They thought of America as a new world dominated by natural behavior, simplicity, and openness—a land unspoiled by the complex societies of Europe. This was far from the truth of course; the Europeans had no awareness of the complexities and conflicts within American society. As the French lionized Franklin as the natural man (an appeal which he lost no time in exploiting), so the English were charmed by Patience's openness, directness with persons, and egalitarianism. Mrs. Adams's harsh judgment of Patience's behavior points up the difference in the way an American and a European would look at her. It also shows the European blindness to the fact that Americans could be as socially conscious as Europeans, despite their more open society. Mrs. Adams was accepted in London society as the ambassador's wife; she surely would not have been if she had acted like Patience. In her position as an American member of an international elite, Mrs. Adams had no reason to accept Patience on equal ground or even make allowances for her, much less idealize her obnoxious behavior. For the Europeans, however, a prominent artist, who counted famous men of both worlds among her friends while being apparently without guile or class consciousness, was something new, and most of all it was something that fit what they wanted to believe about the New World.

They praised her simple manners and her directness in address, her intuitive understanding of people and her dramatic and uninhibited behavior. She seemed to them the embodiment of the democratic spirit of America.

Too, Patience's art coincided with the new trend to realism in English art which was a fresh break with the stilted and conventionalized art long dominated by France. Compared to the correct but lifeless sculpture of the day, Patience's sculptures of living people from all social ranks, lifelike in their detail and color, were wonderfully exciting, seemingly an imitation of nature.

Her critical acclaim in England was based on this. The early announcements of her London wax show in the newspapers lauded her art and later, in 1775, *The London Magazine* devoted a long feature article to her. In it she was praised as "the Promethean modeller" (Prometheus in Greek myth created mankind out of clay), a person of "Integrity, virtue and a pure heart." Her work was described as "a new style of picturing, superior to statuary" and "as perfect as nature."

Patience fit the Europeans' "child of nature" image of Americans, and her art seemed to them the natural expression of such a person. Thus the English overlooked, if they were aware of it (as the English intelligence service certainly was), the anti-British intrigue that composed the other side of her outspokenness, a taste for intrigue that went so far as to propose a ridiculous scheme for revolution in Ireland even after peace was made with England. They overlooked, too, the compulsiveness and distortion of personality that her behavior displayed, a distortion that Watson, an American himself, had noticed in her wild eyes.

PART V

Women Involved Through Their Families

15

Martha Washington

O N THE FIRST DAY of summer in 1731, the first of many children
was born to Colonel John Dandridge and his wife, Frances
Jones. They named the little girl Martha after her maternal grandmother.

By any standard that the New World could offer, the Dandridges
were aristocrats of the first rank. Colonel John was a wealthy planter
whose family reached back to the Dandridges of Great Malvern,
Worcestershire, England, and his wife Frances was a descendant
from a line of scholars and churchmen.

Their estate lay on the banks of the Pamunkey River in New Kent
County just north of Williamsburg, Virginia. Along the Pamunkey
and neighboring York rivers, great mansions with their collections
of stables, mills, shops, and slave quarters spread like small self-
contained towns at the foot of expansive fields of tobacco, grain,
and forage. The larders and smokehouses overflowed with the
robust delicacies of the New World, and even the slaves enjoyed
their meat and fish daily.

Like most of their neighbors in the tidewater region of Virginia,
the Dandridges were forever short of hard cash—their property and
crops being heavily mortgaged to agents in England who provided
them with all the amenities of civilized European life. Wealth,
therefore, was measured in tangible holdings—land, buildings,
slaves, and full storehouses. For the women of these landed estates,
however, wealth and its related social position were measured in
terms of the careful facade of elegance and civilized manners that
hid the tenuous nature of the economy that supported them. Life in
these great houses was not quite as refined as that in London or
even Philadelphia. But the sight of graceful ladies in jewels and silks

moving daintily beneath crystal chandeliers, and the tone of polite conversation emanating from formal drawing rooms were enough to establish Virginian society as a true child of the best that Europe had to offer. Into this world Martha Dandridge was born.

Exactly eight months later at a plantation on Pope's Creek about fifty miles north of the Dandridge estate, Augustine and Mary Ball Washington had a son whom they named George. During the following twenty-six years, the young Washington would distinguish himself as a prominent Virginian gentleman and a gallant soldier, before meeting the young widow of Daniel Parke Custis.

Little is known of the early years of Martha Dandridge, though from her bearing in later life and from a sense of how the young ladies of aristocratic Virginian families were raised, we might reconstruct a picture of her youth.

A quaint early portrait shows her to be of small stature, like all the women in her family—slight, with light brown hair, dark complexion, and hazel eyes. Her education was conducted in the home with emphasis on the skills that she would need to take her place as a wife and mother in Virginian society. She was taught to play the spinet and to dance, but most importantly, she was instructed in the management of a great country house. Apparently mature far beyond her years, Martha's skills in weaving and sewing were developed at an early age and became legendary among her acquaintances. She was schooled in the fine arts of the kitchen, as well as in the preservation and storing of foods, the furnishing and decorating of the house, the planting and harvesting of the kitchen garden, and the supervision of numerous slaves and servants. Above all she was taught the gentle good manners with which such strenuous labor and attention to detail were to be carried out. The most accomplished lady of the manor was no Virginian lady if she lacked the careful graces that were the vehicle for her domestic training.

Of course, Martha was taught to read and write. A young Virginian lady would have to know how to carry on polite correspondence with members of her family and a few close friends, and she would have to be versed in the simple arithmetic necessary for keeping the household accounts. It was a rare woman of the time and place, however, who rose above a level of basic literacy. Her reading consisted of the Bible, sermons and religious tracts, and occasionally, histories and light popular works.

The picture that emerges of these early years is one of a privileged girl of the upper class. But, at its best, eighteenth-century country life in the colonies placed great demands even on the privileged. The title of "mistress" of a plantation house conferred a set of rights and duties that were essential to the maintenance of a way of life. Whatever the wealth of the house and the number of slaves, the task of mistress demanded dedication and special knowledge far beyond any modern concept of housekeeping. Tempered though it was with familial love and the amenities of wealth, the education of Martha Dandridge must have allowed little time for childish frivolity. It was probably this way for most children of her position, boys and girls alike—maintaining a civilized life at the edge of a wild frontier required the intelligence and fortitude that came with thorough training.

In the fall of 1746, Martha Dandridge made her debut into the public life of tidewater Virginia. A few miles to the south of the Pamunkey River lay the capital, Williamsburg, whose well-planned streets and spacious town houses provided an atmosphere of decorum that pleased the Virginians and gave testimony to their growing wealth and confidence. Into the assemblies and balls of this center of law, learning, and society, Martha made her first curtsies.

By all accounts she created a favorable impression from the beginning. She moved gracefully in company, though she avoided the surface gaiety of many of her young fellow patricians, and her conversation was reasonably well-informed and always correct. Her personal grooming was impeccable and the clothes of her own manufacture were models of technical perfection, though modest and conservative. She was immediately noted for her extreme kindness, thoughtfulness, and loyalty to friends, and the parents of eligible bachelors were quick to recognize her considerable domestic talents—as well as the wealth of her family. In those first two years of moving through Virginian society, Martha must have had many interested suitors, though she was too much an example of what Virginia prized most highly in its women for a casual match. Among those she met was Daniel Parke Custis, a bachelor almost thirteen years her senior.

Daniel was the son of Colonel John Custis, one of the wealthiest men in Virginia and master of the White House, an estate on the York River, and the Six-Chimney House, a mansion in Williamsburg. The colonel had advocated the marriage of his son to Evelyn Byrd, the daughter of the rich eccentric, Colonel William Byrd of Westover. Evelyn, however, was several years older than Daniel, and apparently neither entertained much affection for the other. A plodding and reluctant courtship ensued and was finally terminated by the early death of Evelyn.

By the 1740s examples of moderate filial rebellion such as this were not uncommon in the colonies. Almost a century later the French social critic, Alexis de Tocqueville, would note that the roots of American democracy were to be found in the American family. As Daniel Custis and Martha Dandridge were coming of age, the old European-family autocracy was already breaking down in the New World, not because parents were lax or the children defiant and undisciplined, but because the sense of personal liberty and personal responsibility was being extended to include ever larger segments of society. Puritan severity and the patronage system that characterized European aristocratic families were fading in America, where life was less a matter of tradition than a chance for creating new opportunities. It was clear that a young man such as Daniel Custis was free to consider a number of factors, in addition to his father's wishes, while choosing a bride.

Daniel's first consideration, it seems, was purely emotional, for he was immediately taken with the dark smooth complexion, graceful figure, and pleasant manners of Martha Dandridge. Likewise, Martha found Daniel to be the most appealing man in Williamsburg, and the two began a brief courtship. The Dandridge family was well-pleased with the possibilities of this match, and though apparently old Colonel Custis was still nursing some disappointment over the failure of his previous plans for his son, he finally gave his unqualified consent to the marriage.

In June 1749 shortly before her eighteenth birthday, Martha married Daniel Parke Custis at St. Peter's Church in New Kent County. Later that year Colonel John Custis died, leaving Daniel his total estate and the title of colonel. Daniel and Martha had "married well": they were rich and in love and possessed of that enviable feeling that they lived in the best of all possible worlds.

Life for the Custises revolved around their great mansion on the York River and the Six-Chimney House in Williamsburg. They attended all the great balls and dinners, as well as sponsoring many of their own, and the constant round of social visits must have consumed a great deal of their time. Martha wrote no letters to her family during this period, and so it is assumed that she must have visited them often—the Dandridge estate lying only a few miles to the north of the White House.

Within the first five years of marriage, two children were born to the couple, but both died in early childhood. Daniel himself was never in perfect health, though it is doubtful that either he or Martha saw themselves as singled out for a life of personal tragedy. Rampant disease was a fact of life in the eighteenth century and the mortality rate was terrifying by today's standards—especially among children. Usually one could only resort to herbal remedies, purges of one sort or another, or changes of climate. Of course one felt grief at the illness or death of loved ones, though it was rare that such sadness was debilitating in an age when the hold on life was seen as being naturally tenuous.

Within the next three years, Daniel and Martha had two more children who survived. Martha, called Patsy, was born in 1755 and John Parke Custis, called Jacky, in 1757. Shortly after Jacky's birth, in the spring of 1757, Daniel died, apparently of heart failure. After less than eight years of married life, Martha was left a widow at the age of twenty-five.

After Daniel's death Martha and her two children found that they were the sole inheritors, not only of the immense landed estate, but of a sum roughly equivalent to one-half million dollars. This made Martha probably the wealthiest woman, and certainly the wealthiest widow, in all of Virginia. Remaining at the White House, she plunged deeply into her expected period of mourning. Surrounded by her children, her vast entourage, and the sympathetic society of Virginia, Martha's mind must have often wandered to thoughts of the future—her future in a world that placed little value on the half-life of widowhood.

In May 1754 a brief skirmish between a French detachment and a small British colonial army took place at Great Meadows, Pennsylvania, thus initiating the Seven Year's War or, as it is called in America, the French and Indian War. In command of the British troops was Lieutenant Colonel George Washington, then twenty-two years old. In this fight and later on in July at the battle of Fort Necessity, Washington distinguished himself as a brave, albeit amateur, commander. He was promoted to colonel and became something of a hero in the eyes of his fellow Virginians.

Later that same year the king commissioned Governor Horatio Sharpe of Maryland commander of all the British forces. Because Washington was a colonial officer, as opposed to a British officer, this change in command meant that—whatever his rank—he would be subservient to all of the king's officers, even those whom he had previously commanded. Washington's pride ran far too deep to accept this situation, and so in November 1754 he resigned his commission and retired to his home on the Potomac River.

In his will George's father had left him the Ferry Farm plantation near Alexandria, which he was to assume ownership of on his twenty-first birthday. Now, nearing twenty-three, he was still without land, and his aging and increasingly disagreeable mother refused to surrender ownership of the plantation. George's oldest brother, Lawrence, had died willing his plantation, Mount Vernon, to his baby daughter, though she soon died, and the property reverted to his widow. Lawrence's wife remarried, however, and so leased Mount Vernon—with its eighteen resident slaves—to George in perpetuity, for an annual rent of 15,000 pounds of tobacco. In December 1754 George became the squire of Mount Vernon.

Within the year word came from England that a General Braddock was being sent with a large army to further the British cause against the French. With renewed hopes for a military career, George wrote to Braddock upon his arrival and offered his services by reason of his knowlege of the terrain and his experience with Indian fighting. He was immediately accepted on the general's staff and on July 9, 1755 was present at the inglorious defeat of Braddock near Fort Duquesne.

By all accounts—including his own—Washington was a veritable fury on the field of battle and, in recognition, was commissioned a full colonel and commander of all the Virginian forces. Once again the young officer threw himself into the management of a rabble army and the hardships of wilderness warfare.

By March 1758 the long, slow war was beginning to show in George's constitution. He had developed chronic dysentery and his growing weakness forced him to retire to Williamsburg to consult with physicians. It was with a mixture of low spirits and trepidation that he approached the capital.

Having crossed the Pamunkey River with his slave, Bishop, Washington was accosted by a Major Chamberlayne who lived nearby. As was the custom of the day, the major urged George's presence at his table that evening. At first, the young colonel refused, grimly anxious to be off to Williamsburg to hear the verdict of the doctors, but the major pressed him. George left his slave with the horses in front of Chamberlayne's house, determined to take his leave as soon as possible. Once inside he was introduced to the other guests, including the young widow Custis who, now out of mourning, often took refuge here from a growing list of persistent suitors.

After a pleasant dinner, George and Martha found themselves alone in front of one of the great fireplaces, the major and his friends having discreetly retired at an early hour. Toward midnight Bishop was still standing with the horses when a servant notified him that the colonel would be staying the night. The handsome widow and the gallant self-assured officer talked until early morning, George sipping a little wine for the first time in months and perhaps feeling the first blush of returning health.

George continued to Williamsburg the next day where the doctors allayed his fears, prescribing rest and caution in his diet. About one week later, George visited Martha at her own house on the York River, apparently by invitation. After the lavish spread of an early dinner, George and Martha strolled the wide greens of the White House, lost in conversation, bestowing the confidences of old and trusting friends. When George departed that evening, he and Martha were engaged to be married, though they would not meet again until the wedding some nine months later.

By April George had returned to the ranks where a plan was afoot to launch a concerted drive against the French at Fort Duquesne. Through the long summer months of planning and reorganization, George wrote only once to Martha and, in fact, it is his only love letter to her of which we have record. Dated July 20, 1758 at Fort Cumberland, it reads:

> We have begun our march to the Ohio. A courier is starting for Williamsburg, and I embrace the opportunity to send a few words to one whose life is now inseparable from mine. Since that happy hour when we made our pledges to each other, my thoughts have been continually going to you as to another Self. That All-powerful Providence may keep us both in safety is the prayer of your faithful and ever affectionate friend, G. Washington

Plainly, this is not the letter of a passionate fiance, but then it appears that George and Martha were more immensely pleased with one another than they were in love.

Still encamped at Fort Cumberland, Maryland, in September 1758, Washington was making preparations for his coming marriage. George William Fairfax had offered to oversee the readying of Mount Vernon, and an additional story was being added to the house. Martha busied herself with the details of the wedding and made arrangements for transferring the administration of the Custis estate to George.

In November Washington's superior officer, General Forbes, negotiated a treaty with the Indians, who promptly deserted their French allies. George marched on Fort Duquesne to find it burned and abandoned. After arranging for the needs of his men left there in winter camp, the young colonel, who wanted nothing but a military career, resigned his commission and returned to Mount Vernon.

Martha Custis and George Washington were married at the Custis plantation on January 6, 1759. The wedding was an elegant country affair attended by all the notables of tidewater Virginia. Martha was described as wearing a white satin quilted petticoat with heavy corded silk overskirt, shot through with silver threads. Her hair and neck were ornamented with pearls and her high-heeled satin slippers were fastened at the instep with diamond-studded buckles. George wore the full dress of a British officer. The bridal procession traveled to Williamsburg that same day, Martha in a coach drawn by six horses, and George upon his favorite charger. The Washingtons spent their honeymoon at the Six-Chimney House where they remained until early April, when they set out for Mount Vernon.

The mansion had been somewhat enlarged, but it was still smaller and far less opulent than the Custis plantation. Little progress had been made in the years that George had been off fighting the French and neither house nor fields bore the marks of careful attention. The Washingtons faced a considerable challenge in turning Mount Vernon into a home and a plantation that would match their position in Virginian society, but it was a task they both eagerly accepted. It would consume the next fifteen years of their lives.

George became the country squire and gentleman farmer, but he did not act the effete lord of the manor. Riding out into the fields each day, he helped in the draining of swamps and the clearing of new land. He began to diversify his crops and experimented with various grains and forage covers. The land was tilled with new plows of his own design, and mills were built for the grinding of grains and the sawing of lumber.

The task of civilizing Mount Vernon fell to Martha. As a part of her inheritance and dowry, she had brought 150 slaves with her and

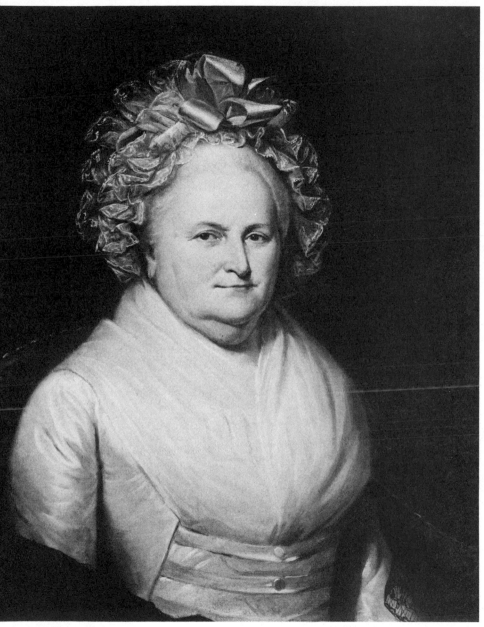

Martha Washington
Courtesy, Independence National Historical Park Collection

now she apportioned them out to various duties. A dairy and smokehouse were put into operation, and as many as thirty-five spinning wheels were kept going at the same time. In a single year, Martha's little factory turned out a total of 1,364 yards of cloth, most of which went for clothing for the slaves since around the house everyone wore homespun. Martha devised and wrote out recipes for the preservation and cooking of foods, as well as such diverse preparations as room deodorants, washing soaps, and even a cleaner and preservative for teeth.

Together Martha and George planned the arrangement of rooms and furnishings: mantelpieces, chandeliers, furniture, and great bolts of silk damasks were ordered from their British agents. All of this cost money, of course, and the price George received for his crops in Europe steadily dropped while the cost of imported goods rose. Most of Martha's inheritance had been consumed in the remodeling and enlargement of Mount Vernon, and by the middle 1760s the Washingtons were back in the position of most Virginian colonials—deeply in debt to London agents who were reluctant to extend further credit.

Nevertheless, George loved to make a fine show, and so the Washington family lived far beyond its means. Martha often accompanied George to Williamsburg to attend the sessions at the House of Burgesses, and she entertained lavishly at the Six-Chimney House. At Mount Vernon George insisted on a continual stream of guests in the best tradition of Virginian gentry, and Martha obliged with groaning tables and an easy domestic charm that often tempted friends and travelers to linger far beyond their intended stay.

George, of course, had adopted Patsy and Jacky as his own and seems to have been greatly fond of them since he and Martha never had any children of their own. Both spoiled the children terribly, though Martha displayed an odd side to her affection. Jacky was left fairly much to his own devices and grew up to be a rather undirected young man, fond of horses and clothes and little else. On the other hand, Patsy, despite her frail disposition, was drilled in the domestic arts much as her mother had been. As was the custom, Patsy was educated in the home while Jack was sent to a school for boys in Caroline County and, at the age of eighteen, entered King's College in New York.

The picture of these years is one of relative ease and happiness for those who, like the Washingtons, could afford it. The French and Indian War had reached its conclusion in 1763, and George's passion for the military had waned as he became more and more involved in the demands of Mount Vernon. By the early 1770s, he had diversified his crops to the point where he was no longer dependent on the foreign market. Actual cash was still lacking, but the Washingtons were solvent enough to enjoy the best that their world had to offer. Between overseeing his farm and expeditions to his newly-acquired holdings in the Ohio valley, George hunted foxes and visited about with his neighbors and old friends, both alone and with Martha. In all, this was a life of civilized domestic sensibility, but it was soon to be rudely interrupted.

In May 1769 the House of Burgesses drew up a resolution proclaiming that it alone, not the British crown, had the right to tax the people of Virginia. Upon receipt of this resolution the royal governor dissolved the House of Burgesses. Most of the members, including Washington, retired to a local tavern and there drew up the charter of the Virginia Non-Importation Association, whose aim it was to refuse the purchase of any taxable item from Britain. Like most of his fellow members, George's loyalty to the British government was still unquestionable and, in fact, that same evening a dinner was held in honor of the queen's birthday.

Martha's attitude toward these developments of the early 1770s seems to have been much the same as her husband's, though she never discussed politics in public except to echo George's sentiments. No doubt she had been as loyal as George, but she was also a Virginian first. When war came, her patriotism to the colonial cause was too active to be passed off as mere wifely subservience. For such an orderly and conservative person, there would need to be great conviction to endure the hardships that lay ahead.

By 1773 little Patsy's health had grown steadily worse, and in June she died in the midst of an epileptic seizure. In a letter to Martha's brother-in-law, George noted that she was " . . . almost reduced . . . to the lowest ebb of misery." To compound her sadness, Jacky had just entered King's College, and so George prevailed upon Martha's mother to take up residence at Mount Vernon. She refused, though early in 1774 Jacky dropped out of college and returned to Virginia, where he married Eleanor Calvert, a member of the prominent Maryland family. Jack and Eleanor moved near

Mount Vernon and this must have been of some comfort to Martha.

If there was a void left behind by these transitions, the Washingtons had little time to reflect on them. In August George was appointed one of the seven Virginian delegates to the first Continental Congress in Philadelphia, and in September he set out with his fellow members, leaving Martha without family in the great house. A colleague of Washington's noted their departure from Mount Vernon.

> I was much pleased with Mrs. Washington and her spirit. She seemed ready to make any sacrifice and was cheerful though I know she felt anxious. She talked like a Spartan mother to her son on going to battle. "I hope you will stand firm—I know George will," she said.

Certainly, Martha foresaw something of the future—the suspension of their comfortable life and the jeopardy into which George's actions would place them—though she noted shortly thereafter in a letter to a relative, "My mind is made up; my heart is in the cause."

The Congress sat for six weeks in Philadelphia, and with customary silence, George listened to the arguments and issues being put forth, absorbing them and deciding on his stand. Upon his return to Virginia, county after county nominated him to lead its militia in the event of war. This ground swell of public sentiment greatly troubled the Washingtons. They found themselves caught between a sense of imminent duty and a fierce protectiveness toward the life they had enjoyed for the past fifteen years. Ultimately, the Washingtons would decide in favor of duty, and though their sacrifice would be made with the greatest reluctance, neither would waver in the difficult years to follow.

In early May 1775, news of the battles at Lexington and Concord reached Mount Vernon. George was immediately elected as a delegate to the second Continental Congress to be held in Philadelphia starting May 10. Once again Martha waved good-bye to her husband and his fellow delegates. George promised to return soon, though he would not see Mount Vernon again—except for two brief visits—for the next eight years.

The talk at the convention centered around two main hopes— that a new, more conciliatory government would come to power in England or that, lacking this, the colonials could stage a brief and successful rebellion that would bring the crown to the negotiating table. For all this talk of rebellion, however, Washington was the sole delegate to the convention who had any technical notions of how the actual warfare might be carried out—should it come to that. When it became clear that the British government would not negotiate, the burden was placed directly on George, and on June 16 he was formally notified that he had been appointed commander in chief of all the colonial armies.

Two days later the general wrote to his wife, breaking the news of his appointment.

> You may believe me, my dear Patsy, when I assure you, in the most solemn manner that, so far from seeking this appointment, I have used every endeavor in my power to avoid it, not only from my unwillingness to part with you and the family, but from consciousness of its being a trust too great for my capacity, and that I should enjoy more real happiness in one month with you at home, than I have the most distant prospect of finding abroad, if my stay were to be seven times seven years.

He went on to say that he could not predict when he would return, though he hoped it would be in the fall. He begged Martha's forgiveness for accepting this responsibility that would so upset their tranquility and gravely noted that he had had a will prepared.

In other letters to Jack and Nelly Custis and to his brother, John, Washington urged them to visit Mount Vernon often and keep Martha company. He also counseled Martha to take up residence farther inland, but she remained at Mount Vernon throughout the war. She would never permit the least decline to set in. All would be kept in constant readiness for the return of her "Old Man," though the long years would drag by without his presence.

In July Washington established his headquarters at Cambridge, outside Boston, in preparation for the first campaign of the war. Throughout that fall the general drove himself and his men to the point of exhaustion in making preparations for the assault on Boston that was planned for the following spring. In November Martha finally received a brief note from George saying that she might come to spend the winter at headquarters, and she set out immediately with her son and his wife.

Soon, however, Martha was shocked to learn that, from Philadelphia northward, the British had spread the rumor that she had been absent from her husband's side for the past seven months because she opposed the American cause and George's commitment to it. Occasional small crowds jeered at her as she passed through Pennsylvania, New Jersey, and New York, though they soon fell silent under her dignified assurances that she was, in fact, no Loyalist. By the time she reached Cambridge in December, the rumors had ceased to have any effect.

In Cambridge the Washingtons celebrated Christmas and their seventeenth anniversary together. Martha set herself to the task of organizing the wives of the other officers, and the knitting of socks and caps and the making of bandages got underway. Throughout that winter Martha acted as assistant secretary to George, copying letters and general orders and keeping the voluminous correspondence from headquarters in order. Despite the cramped quarters of the small house they occupied, Martha always found the time and place to entertain guests, though this seems to have rarely interfered with her work. In a letter to Abigail Adams in the spring of 1776, Mercy Warren noted:

> I took a ride to Cambridge and waited on Mrs. Washington at 11 o'clock, where I was received with that politeness and respect shown in a first interview among the well-bred, and with the ease and cordiality of friendship of a much earlier date. If you wish to hear more of this lady's character, I will tell you I think the complacency of her manners speaks at once of the benevolence of her heart, and her affability, candor, and gentleness qualify her to soften the hours of private life, or to sweeten the cares of the hero, and smooth the rugged paths of war.

Martha must have made a great impression on all who came in contact with her, for from the letters of common foot-soldiers to the diary of Lafayette, all constantly extolled Martha's virtues. She had become a symbol of the gallant, new-American womanhood.

In March 1776 Boston fell to the Americans, and General Washington marched south to set up headquarters in New York. Martha joined him in April, but soon after, the British were sighted off the coast of Cape Cod, and George insisted that she return home. If either George or Martha had entertained hopes that she might remain throughout the campaign, the erratic and unpredictable movements of the British convinced them in the first year that this would be ill-advised. With great sadness Martha set out for Mount Vernon.

On the way south she stopped at Philadelphia where she stayed at the house of John and Dolly Hancock. On the afternoon of July 8, Martha and Dolly heard the pealing of the State House bell signaling the signing of the Declaration of Independence. As crowds cheered in the streets, these two women—who had been privy to the momentous decisions that had led to this event—must have reflected that the ties were now irrevocably severed, that the Americans must win or their own families would be victims of British reprisals. If the American cause should fail, surely George Washington and John Hancock would be hanged as traitors or, at best, spend the rest of their lives in British prisons. Although this thought cast its shadow over the afternoon, both Martha and Dolly felt that special excitement that comes to those who find themselves at a crossroad of great historical implications. Years later Martha would remark with pride that she had heard the first cannon that opened the war at Boston and the last artillery barrage that closed it at Yorktown.

For the next seven years, Martha's life continued the pattern set during this first year of the war. In late fall George would send her notice to join him at winter quarters. Shortly thereafter she would arrive in a simple carriage with a few servants, bringing homespun garments for herself and needed clothes for George. The rest of the carriage would be filled with the delicacies of Mount Vernon which her husband and his fellow Virginians had been denied by the rigors of camp life. For Christmas of each year, at least, the Washingtons shared a great feast.

Throughout each winter Martha and the wives of other officers, as well as many local women pressed into service for the task, would knit and sew for a tattered army that was continually low on provisions. Working the ghastly field hospitals where men lay dying from wounds, disease, and starvation, without medications or even blankets, she would bring whatever cheer she could before returning to her own house where, unseen by others, she would fight back waves of nausea and despair. To her husband, their friends, and that weary little army, however, Martha showed only the face of self-assurance and optimism.

Apparently, few things cheered George more than Martha's arrival. She was his link to the world he so longed to return to, and she, above all others, brought a sense of order and resolve to the dark winter days when his doubts and fears were greatest.

After six years of defeat, starvation, mutiny among the troops, and lack of support from farmers and the populace in general, the colonial armies enjoyed some limited victories and managed to contain the main forces of the British to New York (which the British had retaken in 1776), Charleston, Savannah, and Yorktown, situated by Chesapeake Bay in Virginia. In a surprise move, the French fleet in the West Indies sailed north to effect a blockade of Yorktown, and Washington and Rochambeau marched south to join the small army of Lafayette. To prevent the British forces at New York from sailing to the aid of Lord Cornwallis at Yorktown, these arrangements were carried out with the utmost secrecy. And so with scarcely a day's warning, Washington stopped at Mount Vernon—the first time he had been there since the spring of 1775.

Despite the short notice, Martha's preparations for the visit were elaborate. Comfortable quarters were provided for the general and his staff, and the Mount Vernon kitchens poured forth an abundance of hospitality unequaled during the past six years. For the next three days, Washington, Rochambeau, and Lafayette finalized their plans for the siege of Yorktown, though George was occasionally distracted by the affairs of his house and the four young children of Jack and Nelly Custis whom he had never seen till now. Jack now proclaimed his desire to assist Washington in whatever capacity he might be thought useful, and so he departed with them for Yorktown as George's aide-de-camp.

Cornwallis underestimated his opponents, and through a mixture of brilliant strategy on the part of Washington and Lafayette and, finally, a withering artillery barrage, Yorktown fell to a ragged though determined colonial army. The capitulation was signed on October 19, and a humiliated British army marched out of town.

Before the full joy of this victory could have its effect, however, Jack Custis fell ill with typhus and was removed to the house of a relative some thirty miles from Yorktown. Martha and Nelly were summoned to his side, and on November 5 George arrived just in time to witness Jack's death. George had been looking forward to a few happy days at Mount Vernon, but a pall settled over the house. Martha had lost all her children, Nelly her husband, and George's four stepgrandchildren were fatherless. At the end of the war, George and Martha adopted two of the grandchildren—George Washington Parke Custis and Eleanor Custis, called Nelly after her mother.

George and Martha soon left Mount Vernon for Philadelphia, and there and at Annapolis George received a hero's welcome, though he was often embarrassed by the extreme forms this adulation sometimes took. Throughout Christmas of 1781, George argued with a Congress that was rapidly growing complacent due to the recent great victory. He reminded them that the war was not over yet, and that one significant loss would not necessarily deter the British. With little decided and his army slowly dwindling away, once again George went into winter quarters. Though the last shot of the war had been fired at Yorktown, no clear settlement would be reached for almost two more years. Martha resumed her yearly trek between Mount Vernon and the winter camp, waiting for the end to a war which was already won—if not by complete victory, at least by the reluctance of the British to pursue it.

News of the treaty reached the Washingtons in Princeton at the end of October 1783. Martha returned to Mount Vernon and George took formal possession of New York on November 25. Hurriedly arranging for the dispersal of his army and the return to local control, George rushed toward Annapolis where the Congress was in session. Anxious to resign his commission, he was constantly slowed along the way by banquets and testimonials given in his honor, and he finally reached Annapolis on December 20. Again, three days of balls ensued, and it was not until December 23 that he was allowed to present his formal resignation to the Congress. Riding hard the rest of that day and most of the next, George arrived at Mount Vernon late in the afternoon of Christmas Eve. With the house gaily decorated and a sumptuous feast laid on the table, Martha welcomed George Washington, private citizen—the Virginian gentleman home at last to spend the rest of his days with his family on his beloved plantation.

Life at Mount Vernon settled back into a routine much as it had been before the war. Like Jacky and Patsy before them, the adopted grandchildren, little George and Nelly, demanded a great deal of Martha's time. In all, it seems that the Washingtons' childrearing tactics had changed little in the intervening years—both children were spoiled and doted upon, though Nelly's training was far more rigorous than was George's. In later years they would grow to be much like Martha's own children: Nelly would develop into the perfect aristocratic woman—and would marry well—while George would drop out of King's College after a year of less-than-diligent study. George would try to be stern with the young man in later years, but, basically, both he and Martha were far too infatuated with the children to deny them anything.

Mount Vernon had been loosely managed during George's

absence by his cousin, Lund Washington. Rents had not been collected, debts had piled up with London creditors, and the farm account books were in complete disorder. Once again the Washingtons found themselves land poor, and George would spend the next six years attempting to reestablish the farm as a profit-making enterprise—something at which he never entirely succeeded.

As before, however, the Washingtons never let their technical poverty interfere with their style of living. By the late 1780s, the house had acquired all the trappings of a great Victorian mansion. If anything, the Washingtons now indulged themselves in luxury as never before. If Martha acted to tone down the ostentation that George would have displayed had he free rein, she was no less concerned than he that Mount Vernon be considered a place of absolute comfort and eminent good taste.

If the Washingtons thought that they could regain their old way of life without interruption, however, they were quite mistaken. George's reputation now extended far beyond the boundaries of Virginia. Friends, relatives, neighbors, vaguely-remembered acquaintances, and even sightseers stopped constantly to catch a glimpse of the great general. George was greatly annoyed by these intrusions, though he enjoyed his reputation, perhaps even believing some of the less outrageous attributes that were accorded him. As always, Martha maintained appearances, entertained the guests, and somehow kept order in the midst of confusion. Privately, however, she disliked all the attention—it brought too many strangers to the door, disrupted the careful schedule of the household and, worst of all, threatened the life that she and George had hoped to reclaim out of those long years of war.

By this time Martha must have reflected on the legacy that this fame and the gratitude of the nation would bring them. George insisted that his public life was over, but it was clear that he had been too much a part of the events that initiated the birth of the new nation to be allowed to retire into obscurity. In fact, he took a great interest in the affairs of the nation. Throughout the 1780s, as Congress attempted to govern the independent states through the Articles of Confederation, he often wrote letters to various friends and delegates, commenting on issues and offering recommendations. On several occasions he was urged to use his influence to work out disputes, though he always declined in favor of the demands of his plantation.

By early 1787 severe problems that seemed to indicate the need for a stronger government prompted Congress to call for a special convention to revise the Articles of Confederation. Promptly elected as presiding officer, Washington's great influence soon came to bear on what revealed itself as the true purpose of the convention. Rather than revise the Articles, a new constitution was written and sent to the separate states for ratification.

Though Washington declined to discuss it in any but the most oblique terms, this document provided for a president to head the Executive Branch, and it was generally assumed in Congress that the first president could only be one man. Because of this near-unanimous support, George knew that his refusal could seriously endanger the success of the new government, though he kept to himself about this, awaiting the final outcome of the state conventions.

By July 1788 the required number of states had ratified the Constitution, and the starting date for the new government was set for March of the following year. That February the electors met in their respective states and cast their ballots for president. On April 14 the secretary of Congress rode up to Mount Vernon to inform George Washington that he had been elected the first president of the United States.

Martha was not present on April 30 when George was inaugurated in New York, nor was she present for the great reception ball that followed. There had never been a president or a president's wife before, and lacking any sense of protocol and etiquette appropriate to the station, George had her delay at Mount Vernon until such decisions were made. In a frenzy of invention, Adams, Hamilton, and Jay designed a basic schedule of appointments and social functions that would regulate the daily affairs of both the presidential office and the president's household. Finally, a large renovated house was leased for the Washingtons.

Some semblance of order having been created in New York, George sent for his wife and family. Martha arrived in New York on May 28 with the two adopted grandchildren and seven black and fourteen white servants. Within three days Martha held the first of her "levees"—social receptions for the elite of the town—and by this time had laid aside her homespun garments in favor of the more elegant dress of city society.

At Mount Vernon and during the war it had been necessary to be merely clean and neat, except at formal entertainments. Now

Martha had to present a daily show—something that ran counter to the habits of her past life. She kept her sense of humor about this, though. In a letter to a niece, shortly after her arrival in New York, she wrote, " . . . my hair is set and dressed every day—and I have put on white muslin habits for the summer—you would I fear think me a good deal in the fashion if you could but see me. . . . "

Martha now found herself in another new situation with new adjustments to make at an age when she would rather have been quietly keeping her own house. Her dissatisfaction, carefully disguised in public, must have added a gravity to her demeanor which others took as further evidence of her already-awesome dignity. Whatever her feelings, the old Virginian training and an uncompromising sense of duty would carry Martha through again.

The Washingtons moved almost immediately to a larger, more fashionable house near Bowling Green, which the government leased for them at the then outrageous sum of $2,500 per year. In addition to the family and the servants, George's personal secretaries lived in the same house, and a social round began such as had not been seen even during the most hectic days at Mount Vernon. George held his levees at the house on Tuesdays and Martha held hers on Fridays. An official dinner was given each Thursday, and there were guests for dinner and conversation afterward each night. Under the new etiquette, the Washingtons were to have Sunday evenings to themselves, though even then a few close friends were always invited.

The dinners at the house on Bowling Green were mostly formal with huge amounts of food, but George would never sample more than one dish at a sitting, taking along with it one pint of beer and two glasses of wine. He would rarely sit with the men more than fifteen minutes after the ladies had retired; he would then join Martha and the ladies for coffee in the drawing room. These dinners were generally considered to be the dullest affairs in town: George made little conversation and seemed mostly preoccupied. In deference to him the others would also maintain silence, broken only occasionally by the pressing affairs of state or embarrassed attempts at levity.

Conversation went somewhat better in the drawing room owing to Martha's expert direction, though even here the old country charm was lacking. Under her stiff brocades and the oppressive sense of formality and decorum, Martha did not know—in fact, had no way of knowing if she was behaving properly for the wife of a president. The truth was that, even in the society of New York, which was so preoccupied with correct form, no one had any good idea how the president and his lady should behave. Throughout this first year, the New York newspapers would continually gossip about the Washingtons' sense of style or lack of same.

Since the custom of the president's wife being exempt from the responsibility of paying personal calls was not yet established, Martha promptly returned visits from the wives of friends and officials on the third day, arriving in a coach with four horses and preceded by a footman who announced her arrival. She attended to charities—both she and George giving heavily to individuals and organizations—and on Sundays she attended Trinity Church, either alone or with her husband. Except for formal entertainments, she still dressed as plainly as her station would allow, and usually wore no jewelry other than a simple locket containing a miniature of George and a lock of his hair. Apart from the brief hours of seclusion between the time she went to bed and her early rising at 5:30, Martha bore the strain of constant social obligation, engaging in careful conversation, nodding assent to the Federalist cause, forcing politeness to members of the opposition, and taking care to refer to George as "the general" or "the president" where before she had always openly called him "Papa."

Despite her previous resolve to face this new life with a cheerful attitude, a later note to Fanny Washington, the wife of George's favorite nephew, revealed either a wishful exaggeration or a momentary break with her obligations:

I live a very dull life here and know nothing that passes in the town—I never goe to any publick place—indeed I think I am more like a state prisoner than anything else, there is certain bounds set for me which I must not depart from—and as I cannot doe as I like I am obstinate and stay home a great deal.

It is doubtful that Martha ever acted the complete recluse; her sense of duty and growing confidence would not let her.

In August 1790 Congress acted to establish a new capital city for the nation, at a location to be chosen by Washington on the banks of the Potomac near Georgetown. In the interim the capital was to be moved to Philadelphia as a concession to the politicians there. Neither George nor Martha had been overly fond of New York, and now they prepared to leave as soon as the arrangements for the move could be made. After a brief stay at Mount Vernon, they went to Philadelphia where they would remain for the next six years.

Urged on once again by his friends in the Congress and by his cabinet, Washington accepted the bid for president and was reelected in 1793. He was the only person with enough popularity nationwide to hold the young government together, and it was for this reason that he accepted the nomination, though it meant that another four years stood between Martha and him and the longed-for life as private citizens back at Mount Vernon.

The new government was picking up momentum under George's cautious leadership, but overwhelming problems remained. To further complicate matters, George's popularity among the politicians began to wane somewhat as the number and intensity of factions increased. He was accused of secret ambitions to become a monarch, and the elegant style of living that the Washingtons adopted in Philadelphia was criticized constantly by the Republican and other opposition presses.

In fact, it is doubtful that George ever entertained any kingly notions, though he had become short-tempered and haughty, especially with his critics who advocated a mass, popular democracy as opposed to a system of strong central government. He had personally abhorred the rise of factional politics, and now that he found himself powerless to prevent it, he withdrew into his old aristocratic Virginian ways. Here he was on firm ground, living a life that he thought most appropriate to a man of his station.

Surprisingly, Martha was no less responsible than George for the courtly appearance that their life had assumed. She had begun to adapt to the idea of being the first lady of the land, and as their status increased and the etiquette of the presidential office grew more complex, so too the simple Virginian housewife turned herself out with a grander show than she ever had previously. Her dress took on more of the look popular in Philadelphia high fashion. Instead of a plain chariot, she now went out in a coach described as being in the shape of a hemisphere, ornamented with cupids, supporting festoons, and with borderings of flowers around the panels. Dinners at the High Street mansion became models of American gastronomic opulence.

Despite the many balls, frequent evenings at the theater, and her own newly-found willingness to engage in a more active social life, Martha remained steadfast in her views of what constituted acceptable society and proper behavior. If she found greater comfort and happiness in Philadelphia, it was because she acquired many close friends—none of whom were members of the ultra-fashionable group of the town. She complained that most of the Philadelphia elite were given to shallow and excessive gaiety, and the majority of social events were tedious exercises in superficial manners. Martha would accompany George about town as duty demanded, but she would reserve her own drawing room and her best social graces for that close circle of intimates.

Martha remained above politics as she always had in the past, even now in the intense atmosphere of factional disputes that plagued Washington's second administration. To be sure, few anti-Federalist Democrats or Republicans ever graced her drawing room, but her objections to them seem to have had more to do with manners than political beliefs.

The war and the transfer of power from British to American hands had contributed to a growing class of gentry—and pretenders to gentry—in the United States. Merchants, military officers, and a proliferating number of government officials and bureaucrats had managed to extract profit and fame from patriotism and were steadily moving into the upper strata of society. With their obscure family origins and coarse manners, they would buy or bully their way into the circles of the old aristocracy, and Martha found their presence thoroughly unwelcome. As it happened, many of them were also affiliated with that democratic, common-man orientation that saw old dangers in the strong central government of "King" George Washington.

The only vicious thing that Martha was ever known to have said, probably the only time she lost her poise in public, concerned her impatience with these "new" Americans. One afternoon, her grand-daughter Nelly was supposed to be practicing on the harpsichord, but instead was entertaining a would-be suitor. At the sound of Martha's approach the young man fled, leaving a smudge from his oily hair on the wall above the settee. "Ah, it was no Federalist," exclaimed Lady Washington. "None but a filthy Democrat would mark a place with his good-for-nothing head in that manner!" Martha's concern seems to have been centered more on the social *faux pas,* however, than on the young man's political leanings. We may be sure that none of Martha's friends ever left a blemish on her drawing room walls, whatever their politics.

Throughout the remaining years in Philadelphia, Martha entertained a great deal in private and, when the affairs of state impinged on their domestic life, she provided that tasteful ambience for which the Washington household became well-known. The older children of Nelly Custis visited often, and several of the Washingtons' nieces and nephews stayed with them for extended periods of time. On family evenings the young people would hold informal dances, stepping out the Virginia Reel, with George often coming out of his study to join in. These must have been the most treasured evenings for the Washingtons for they recreated a bit of the atmosphere of Mount Vernon.

Formal dinners were a constant occurrence, and in addition to the heads of state and other notables, Washington was fond of inviting large parties of Indian chiefs and their wives to dine. There is no record of Martha's attitude toward having these envoys of the wilderness at her elegant tables, though others often viewed George's paternalism with amusement. It was, however, less a matter of paternalism than a deep concern for the Indians which Washington, in the semi-enlightened atmosphere of Philadelphia, could deal with more openly than the real burning issue of the time—that of slavery. Accordingly, Indians dined at his table, and their problems were discussed while blacks served the food.

Washington was personally opposed to slavery, but he was well aware of the attitudes of his fellow southerners and refused to make an issue of it during his administration. His opposition, of course, was one in principle. As an owner of slaves who worked his numerous farms, he had private interests to protect, though in his will he provided for the freeing of all his slaves upon the death of Martha. In later years it was charged that, eager for their liberty, the slaves hurried her demise, and on the basis of this rumor James Madison changed his will which had read the same as George's. This is doubtful, however, for the Washingtons had always been relatively liberal with their slaves, though an incident in 1792 shows that Martha was still of an old-fashioned Virginian mind. Her personal servant of many years, a slave woman named Oney, ran away and headed, it was thought, for Canada. Very much incensed, Martha demanded that George advertise throughout New England for her return. George declined, noting that it would not look quite right for the president of an egalitarian republic to advertise for a runaway slave, but Martha was not to be mollified in the face of Oney's "ingratitude."

During the eight years of his presidency, Washington had literally created the office out of the abstract concept delineated in the Constitution. In retrospect it appears that he was probably the only man in America with the particular talents and wide appeal to make it work, and though his second administration ended without complete solutions for severe foreign and domestic problems, he would leave behind a firmly established government and a strong presidential office which would serve the needs of the country for a long time to come.

In 1796 Washington was approached again and asked to run for a third term in office, but now he finally refused. He had served his country in one capacity or another for forty-five years, he was nearing sixty-seven years of age, and now his single desire was to return to Mount Vernon. He also foresaw the possible dangers of accepting a third term—it would further divide the nation by lending some credence to the charges that he was fast becoming a monarch, and it could establish an unwelcome precedent that might prove problematic in the future. Good judgment and not a little fatigue combined, and George resolutely looked forward to his retirement. By January 1797 Adams had been elected the new president and, after completing his last official acts, Washington arranged for the departure of his family from Philadelphia.

Shortly after their arrival at Mount Vernon, Martha wrote an old friend:

> I cannot tell you . . . how much I enjoy *home* after having been deprived of one for so long, for our dwelling in New York and Philadelphia was not *home,* only a sojourning. The General and I feel like children just released from school or from a hard taskmaster, and we believe that nothing can tempt us to leave the sacred roof tree again, except on private business or pleasure. We are so penurious with our enjoyment that we are loath to share it with anyone but dear friends, yet almost every day some stranger claims a portion of it, and we cannot refuse. I am again settled down to the pleasant duties of an old-fashioned Virginia housekeeper, steady as a clock, busy as a bee, and cheerful as a cricket.

Martha's "lost days," as she always referred to the years in public life, were finally over, but even now absolute privacy was to be denied to her and George. During the last twenty years they had had only two dinners alone together, and now Nelly Custis, the other grandchildren, several nieces, and the young son of Lafayette and his tutor were all living at the mansion. George hired a permanent housekeeper to ease Martha's burden, and, except for close friends, the Washingtons left their guests more and more to their own devices, often visiting them only at tea and dinner.

Nevertheless, a great amount of work needed to be done at Mount Vernon and the Washingtons tried to pick up where they had left off eight years earlier. George resumed his old tasks of renovating and adding on to the house and outbuildings, spending most of his days in the fields, overseeing his mills and fisheries and expanding the number of acres under cultivation.

For her part, Martha's ceaseless industry continued though constant demands were placed on her time by the arrival of curious strangers. She still rose at dawn, and after breakfast she would retire to her chamber to spend an hour reading the Scriptures and praying. At her entertainments friends noted that she was still the perfect hostess, giving all her attention to the comfort and well-being of her guests. Now her conversation reflected the wealth of experience she had accumulated since the beginning of the war. She recalled old friends and great events, and compared at length the current administration with that of her husband—often, these days, with a certain acidity and sarcasm reserved for the likes of Jefferson and his fellow Republicans.

In the last year of his life, George found even less time to spend on his plantation. War threatened from the new government of France, and he was pressed to resume his role as commander of the American armies. Ultimately, war was never declared and no French troops ever set foot on American soil, but throughout the fall of 1798 and spring of 1799 Washington poured his energies into the reorganization of the army. Back at Mount Vernon financial problems grew, and for the first time in his life George had to take out a bank loan. Torn between duty to his country and his passionate desire to be left alone to his farming, Martha's old man never found the peace he had hoped for in his last years.

On December 12, 1799 Washington rode out as usual to inspect his farm. The weather was dreadful and by the time he returned, he had sat astride his horse for five hours in driving rain, hail, and snow. Snowflakes were frozen to his hair when he entered the house, and his secretary mentioned that he appeared soaked. George dismissed this and retired early, but he awoke the next morning with a sore throat. By midnight he could barely speak and was breathing with difficulty, though he refused aid, saying, "Let it go as it came." That day the doctor was called and the usual bleedings and other remedies were tried, but by the evening of December 14 George was in severe pain, gasping for short breaths. About ten o'clock Martha looked up from the foot of the bed where she sat; the slight movement of the cover over her husband's chest had ceased. "Is he gone?" she asked calmly. Overcome by tears, the doctor ineffectually raised his hand in assent. "'Tis well," she said in the same even voice. "All is over now; I shall soon follow him; I have no more trials to pass through."

George was buried two days later at Mount Vernon, but within the week Congress sent a letter to Martha requesting that she give her permission for the removal of the president's remains to a tomb in the new capital city of Washington. Even now, possibly the saddest moment of her life, her reply was characteristic. It read in part:

> Taught by the great example which I have so long before me never to oppose my private wishes to the public will—I must consent to the request made by congress. . . .

Washington's body was never moved, however, but was eventually interred in a vault which he had designed at Mount Vernon. It was here, at a place near the house called the Vineyard Enclosure, that Martha came daily, not to mourn, but to recall the fantastic memories of a full life.

In accordance with the custom of closing the death chamber for three years, their bedroom was sealed and Martha moved into a small attic room directly above. From the dormer windows she could look out on her husband's grave, and there she spent much of her time for the next two years, surrounded by her knitting, servants, and ever-present friends and relatives. Sometime in her last year, she burned all of the letters George had written to her over the past forty years. She must have realized that all of her husband's records and documents would receive the greatest attention in the years to come. As a loyal and discreet friend to the last, she would not allow his intimacies and secrets to be subjected to public scrutiny.

On May 22, 1802, on the seventeenth day of a severe fever, Martha requested the last sacraments from her minister. Calling for the white gown she had laid aside for the occasion, she spoke in a strong voice to her assembled grandchildren and other relatives concerning the great value of religion, the need for attention to practical duties, and the absolute importance of doing well for others. Her sermon finished and her bedclothes neatly arranged, she lay back on her pillow and closed her eyes. A few hours later, at noon, she died quietly in her sleep.

16

Sarah Franklin Bache

BENJAMIN FRANKLIN'S DAUGHTER Sarah was an author and a relief worker during the Revolution. While her father was abroad, she also served as hostess to the important Europeans to whom he gave letters of introduction. Among her guests were Thomas Paine and the French minister, Conrad Alexandre Gerard. The considerations she showed her guests on behalf of the Patriots' cause impressed them deeply and may have contributed to the generosity of foreign assistance to the war effort.

Sarah Bache is most remembered for her relief work. She was among the organizers led by Esther de Berdt Reed to raise money for General Washington's army and was one of five members of the executive committee, sharing the leadership of the ladies' association with Mrs. Reed. Joseph Reed was at this time the chairman of the committee of local Patriots which governed Philadelphia. When Mrs. Reed died in 1780, the very year the work was begun, Sarah Franklin Bache became the moving force on the executive committee that remained. Sarah had herself contributed 400 continental dollars to the work, one hundred of which were given on behalf of her daughter Elizabeth.

Finally, the proposed sum was collected. Acting upon Washington's suggestion, the executive committee used the money to purchase cloth to make shirts for the soldiers of the Continental army. Then Sarah's talents for persuasion were put to a great test—to convince the good ladies of Philadelphia that they had not already done enough, and that they must participate in the manufacturing of shirts.

The shirts were cut out in Sarah's home, with her household contributing most heavily to the effort. The picture of the most elegant women of Philadelphia gathered in a great hall to make shirts for the most lowly soldiers in the Continental army excited the minds of European visitors. The highest society in London or Versailles would never be engaged in such lowly work. The social responsibility felt by these leaders of American society was one unique feature of this land. The Marquis de Chastellux even interrupted his travels in America to visit the workrooms and wrote an account of what he found in this journal entry of December 1, 1780:

> She conducted us into a room filled with needlework, recently finished by the ladies of Philadelphia. This work consisted neither of embroidered tambour waistcoats, nor network edging, nor of gold or silver brocade—but of shirts for the soldiers of Pennsylvania. The ladies had bought the linen from their own private purses, and had gladly cut out and stitched the shirts themselves. On each shirt was the name of the married or unmarried lady who made it, and there were 2,200 shirts in all.

After such an account of the virtue and patriotism of the ladies of Philadelphia, Chastellux felt compelled to defend the same qualities in Frenchwomen. He was sure that if the French were in similar circumstances, their women would inspire the same kind of account.

On December 26, 1780, Sarah Franklin Bache informed General Washington that the ladies had completed the shirts which were ready for delivery to the army. Immediately after delivery letters in praise of his daughter were received by Benjamin Franklin in France. "The Ladies concerned in this affair, have gained immortal honour, of which Mrs. B. might claim a capital share," wrote Isaac All, a ship's captain married to a cousin of Sarah's. French officers in America were even more extravagant in their praise of Sarah's work. In a letter to Benjamin Franklin written almost a year after the shirts were finished, M. de Marbois spoke of the efforts on behalf of the soldiers. He felt the ladies of Philadelphia could have instructed their European sisters in domestic virtue and patriotism.

> If there are in Europe any women who need a model of attachment to domestic duties and love for their country, Mrs. Bache may be pointed out to them as such. She passed a part of last year in exertions to rouse the zeal of the Pennsylvania ladies, and she made on the occasion such a happy use of the eloquence which, you know, she

possesses, that a large part of the American army was provided with shirts bought with their money or made by their hands. In her application for this purpose, she showed the most indefatigable zeal, the most unwearied perseverance, and a courage in asking, which surpassed even the obstinate reluctance of the Quakers in refusing.

Benjamin Franklin could be all the more proud of his daughter because she was a perfect example of the results to be achieved when his ideas of education were followed. Sarah's early schooling had been better than that of most American women of the time. In addition to reading and writing, she was instructed in arithmetic, needlework, dancing, French, and music. Any skill in which she had been instructed was maintained throughout her life, and Francis Hopkinson said in 1785 when Sarah was more than forty, that she played the harpsichord "very well." She had also practiced at the armonica, a musical instrument of her father's invention.

Benjamin Franklin acquired such a high opinion of his daughter that very early he began to be concerned about the identity of her future husband. In correspondence with his friend William Strachan, he only half joked about an arranged marriage. A letter from Franklin on June 21, 1750 contained his description of his daughter, under a guise of the suggestion that she at seven be engaged to Strachan's son at ten.

> I am glad to hear so good a Character of my Son-in-Law. Please acquaint him that his spouse grows finely, and will probably have an agreeable Person. That with the best Natural Disposition in the World, she discovers daily the Seeds and Tokens of Industry, Oeconomy, and in short every Female Virtue, which her Parents will endeavor to cultivate for him; and if Success answer their fond Wishes and Expectations, she will in the true sense of the Word, be *worth* a great deal of Money, and consequently a great fortune.

After another seven years, Franklin was still writing in this vein, referring to "our son Billy" Strachan (then seventeen) and "our Daughter Sally" (then fourteen). In 1760 the Strachan family formally proposed a marriage between Sarah and William. Benjamin accepted the proposal under the condition that his wife, Deborah, take up permanent residence in England with the couple.

It was one of the severest trials of Franklin's life that he was in England when his daughter's courtship by Richard Bache was begun and brought to fruition. His first reaction to the news was contained in a letter to Deborah written in May 1767.

My Love to Sally: In answer to what was written to me by you, and by her, and Mr. Bache, I wrote particularly to every one by Mr. Odell, that I left the Matter to you and her Brother, for at this Distance I could neither make any Enquiries into his Character and Circumstances, nor form any Judgement, And as I was in doubt whether I should be able to return this Summer, I could not occasion a Delay of her Happiness if you thought the Match a proper one.

By the end of the summer, Benjamin was less willing to leave the decision to his wife, since he had news of a reversal in the affairs of Mr. Bache. So in August he wrote two letters which he expected would delay if not prevent the match. In the first he advised the young man to wait to marry Sarah until his situation was improved. In his letter to Deborah he seemed to expect that the young suitor's decision to stall marriage plans was an accomplished thing.

In your last Letters you say nothing concerning Mr. Bache. The misfortune that has lately happened to his Affairs, tho' it may not lessen his Character as an honest or prudent Man, will probably induce him to forbear entering hastily into a State that will require a great Addition to his expence, when he will be less able to supply it.

Contrary to Benjamin Franklin's expectations of caution, twenty-four-year-old Sarah Franklin married Richard Bache on October 29, 1767. The ships in Philadelphia's harbor celebrated the marriage of the prominent couple by breaking out their colors the next day. Jane Mecom sent a letter of congratulations to her brother, Benjamin Franklin, speaking highly of a match he did not yet approve.

For several months after he learned of the marriage, Benjamin Franklin did not correspond with his daughter and her new husband. When finally he did write in August of 1768, he was not much more positive about the match than he had been in silence. But Sarah was overjoyed by the resumption of communication with her father.

Richard Bache's finances improved till he was once again among the most important merchants of Philadelphia. When finally the father and son-in-law met in 1771, Franklin liked the choice his daughter had made and permitted the young family to live rent free in part of the Franklin family complex of two houses that were constructed so as to meet in the middle.

Sarah's life for the next few years revolved around the nursery where she kept eight children, of whom seven survived childhood.

She once apologized that as the daughter of a national figure she yet knew "very little that passed out of the nursery, where indeed it is my greatest pleasure to be." Her last child was born in 1788, almost twenty years after her first, but she did not spend those more than twenty years occupied solely with the nursery.

The Revolutionary War changed Sarah Bache's life in a variety of ways. Her husband was appointed postmaster general in 1776 and was often away from home and in danger of capture. In that same year, her father took her eldest son to France, where the child remained to be educated until 1785. Sarah was also forced to move her household to avoid the thrust of British forces. When the British officers advanced through New Jersey in 1776, Sarah took refuge in Goshen, Chester County. Very far advanced in pregnancy, Sarah bore her second daughter in Goshen. Four days after childbirth, Sarah again gathered up her household and fled to Lower Dublin Township and then to Manheim, Pennsylvania. After all of this effort and the terror and exhaustion of giving birth in flight, Sarah resolved to stay with her family in Philadelphia next time the British advanced.

Deborah Franklin died in 1774 after a wasting illness. Following the death of her mother, Sarah became the head of her father's household in America and an even more important figure in Philadelphia as the importance of Benjamin's French connections grew during the war. She wrote frequent and detailed letters to her father complaining of the inflation and meager supply of ordinary commodities. She announced in one letter that she had to send her maid to market with two baskets—one to carry the piles of money required to buy the day's victuals and the other to carry home the supplies.

> There is hardly such a thing as living in town, everything is so high, the money is old tenners to all intents and purposes. If I was to mention the prices of the common necessities of life, it would astonish you. I have been all amazement since my return; such an odds have two years made that I can scarcely believe I am in Philadelphia.

This letter had been written at the beginning of the new social season when the returning Patriots and welcome strangers celebrated the recapture of the city. In her letters Sarah mentioned having met General and Mrs. Washington at several parties. By return

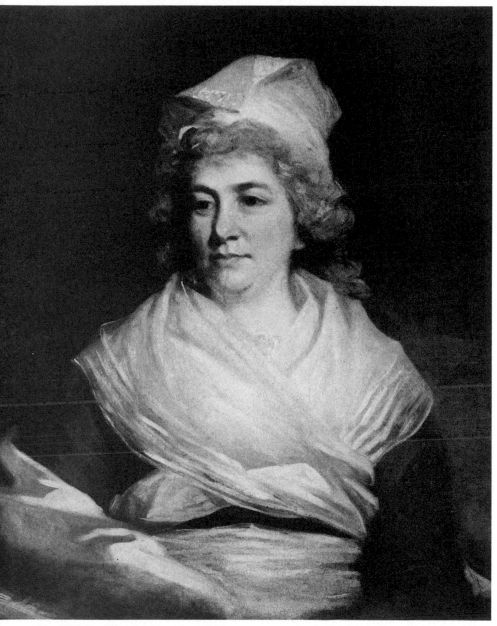

Sarah Franklin Bache (Portrait by John Hoppner)
Courtesy, The Metropolitan Museum of Art, Wolfe Fund, 1901

letter Benjamin Franklin expressed his feeling that the gaiety was unseasonable. He was concerned lest the French believe no more assistance on their part would be necessary to ensure victory. Sarah offered a different perspective on the season.

> But how could my dear papa give me so severe a reprimand for wishing a little finery. He would not, I am sure, if he knew how much I have felt it. Last winter was a season of triumph to the Whigs, and they spent it gaily. You would not have had me, I am sure, stay away from the Ambassador's or General's entertainments, nor when I was invited to spend the day with General Washington and his lady; and you would have been the last person, I am sure, to have wished to see me dressed with singularity. . . . I can assure my dear papa that industry in this country is by no means laid aside; but as to spinning linen, we cannot think of that til we have got that wove which we spun three years ago.

She later on declared with pride that her husband could not bear to be merchandising under the present conditions of monopoly and excess profit.

Sarah Franklin Bache was her father's hostess from the time of his return to Philadelphia in 1785 until his death in 1790. She presided over the great doctor's tea table while her young children whirled about her skirts. Washington called several times in the summer of 1787 and gave to Sarah a copy of Joel Barlow's *Vision of Columbus* as he was leaving the city.

Following her father's death, Sarah sold some diamonds encrusting a miniature which had been presented to her father by King Louis XIV of France. With the proceeds of this sale, Sarah took most of her family to England, where she was hailed as the toast of the season by a society which had admired her father. This journey was undertaken in 1792 when Sarah was almost fifty.

The most interesting incident of her later years was reported by her grandchildren. Apparently some of her children were attending a school where the headmistress wished to seat her pupils according to the social rank of their parents. Upon hearing of this seating arrangement, "Mrs. Bache sent her word that in this country there was no rank but rank mutton." Another example of their grandmother's wit was likewise reported by these biographers. "One night, upon sitting up in bed, she spied a rat eating the candle on the mantel. She aroused her husband, who said sleepily, 'My dear, there is no rat, it is conceit.' 'Very well, Mr. Bache, then it is conceit with four legs and a tail.'" As sleepy as he was, the poor man slew the rat, being no match for his wife's wit.

In her later years, Sarah was surrounded by affectionate family and friends. She became ill with cancer and died in October 1808 at the age of sixty-four.

17

Catherine Littlefield Greene

CATHERINE LITTLEFIELD GREENE was the wife of General Nathaniel Greene, who was second only to George Washington in his contributions to American victory during the Revolutionary War. She was valued by the ragged troops at Valley Forge and by the most sophisticated society of America for her spontaneous gaiety and personal warmth. She contributed to the American cause through her tenacious support for her husband and her willingness to alleviate despair by sharing the privations of war. In her lifetime she bonded revolutionary courage to the striving ingenuity of the new American character.

Born February 17, 1755 in New Shoreham, Rhode Island, on Block Island, Catherine Littlefield was her parents' first daughter and the third of five children. The Littlefields had come to Rhode Island from Massachusetts earlier in the century. Her father married the daughter of one of New Shoreham's oldest families and served in the colonial assembly from 1747 until the beginning of the War for Independence.

Little is known of Kitty's childhood. Like most of the children in New Shoreham, she attended the town school, learning the basic skills and a few graces but not much more. She was a member of the Baptist meetinghouse in the little fishing and farming community. Her life on Block Island revealed little of her future until she was old enough to visit her mother's prominent family connections in Rhode Island's more populous areas.

Most important of all influences on the very young Kitty Littlefield was her friendship with the aunt after whom she had been named. Catherine Ray Greene's husband was active in Rhode Island politics and would later be the state's second governor. The

Greenes were close friends with Benjamin Franklin and maintained correspondence with him whether he was at home or abroad. It was through her Aunt Catherine that Kitty met the man she was to marry, Nathaniel Greene, a distant kinsman from Coventry, Rhode Island.

When Catherine met Nathaniel Greene, he was a comfortably established and popular bachelor in his early thirties. With his one living brother, he shared an inheritance of several well-run saw and grist mills and a prosperous forge. The Greene family had been prominent Quakers in Rhode Island for five generations. Greene had built for himself a large and comfortable home in Coventry, overlooking the Narragansett Bay across from Newport. With a guaranteed substantial living from family businesses, he was considered a very eligible bachelor.

It was probably not so much Nathaniel's property which attracted young Kitty's attention as it was his social polish. Nathaniel Greene had educated himself in philosophy, military history, and literature, to the great discomfort of his family who felt that he only needed knowledge of the Bible and enough arithmetic to calculate accounts. Though the family was well enough off to provide for the young man's education, he had to purchase books with spending money earned by fashioning toys at the forge as a child. Because Nathaniel was a hard worker and competent manager at the forge, his father indulged him by letting him go to a little Latin school in East Greenwich for a short time when he was fourteen. His family gave no consideration to his needs for time to study, so he read while attending to the fires and hoppers at the grist mill. His brother reported years later that young Nat had to absent himself from the family hearth and remain in a cold and poorly lighted upstairs room in order to study in the evening. The knowledge which Nathaniel Greene acquired from his books later gained him acceptance into the most graceful circle of Newport's elegant society. In the colonies educated men were accorded a certain social prominence, regardless of the irregular fashion in which they had obtained their knowledge.

Even as a very young Quaker, Nathaniel Green had eschewed the severity of outlook shared by his father and most of the brethren. He had frequently broken his father's curfew by sneaking out for clandestine meetings with young friends, returning to the sure punishment of his parents when the mischief was over. Though he dressed as a Quaker, Greene did so with more than the accustomed polish. His drab suit of clothes was smartly tailored for him by a prominent Boston merchant. The broad-rimmed hat, customarily worn by all Quaker men, was often purchased during Greene's excursions to Boston. Nathaniel enjoyed parties and large social events. He even danced, though poorly because of a limp from childhood. With his education, his laboriously acquired polish, and the Quaker trait of humility, Nathaniel Greene was an attractive addition to any guest list in Newport or Providence.

The boys with whom Nat Greene had played mischievously as a youth became the most important figures in a growing debate over dissatisfaction with British rule. James Varnum and Samuel Ward were only a few of his close friends who were forming local volunteer companies and sending petitions and letters throughout the colonies. Nathaniel Greene's library had grown from the few classics he could afford in his youth. It now encompassed the latest works of literature and enlightenment philosophy, which were firing colonial intellectuals with high ideals about the inherent rights of men and the nature of the social contract. As discontent grew, Greene shared in worried and serious conferences with his fellows. Soon he began to espouse the un-Quaker-like policy of armed resistance to tyranny if the British Parliament did not desist. This gave him an unsatisfactory reputation for a Quaker, and his assembly did not blink at his attitude.

If the Quaker assembly was dismayed by Nathaniel Greene's reputation as a firebrand, Kitty Littlefield was not. Nathaniel Greene was to her young eyes the most exciting of all the men she had met in the elegant world beyond Block Island. Kitty was a bubbly young woman with just enough family background and polish to be accepted at the elegant balls and soirées of Newport and Providence. She was delightfully aware of the effect her youthful vibrance had on Nat Greene. Soon they began planning their wedding for late July 1774.

Before Nathaniel Greene took Kitty to the ample home he had built in Coventry, he was already certain that political events would occupy his next few years. During the summer of 1774 while preparing to receive a new wife into his bachelor's home, Nathaniel Greene began to put into practice his readings in military history and discipline. He was one of the first volunteers to the newly formed independent volunteer companies called the Kentish Guards. All the members of the company were his childhood companions and now prominent citizens. The time had come to choose sides, Greene felt, and he was unsure of Kitty's reaction should he choose the hazardous course of rebellion against the crown. He need not have worried; Kitty was as enraged at British interference in colonial rights as he was. After all, she was preparing for her wedding while living in Aunt Catherine's home, which was anxiously preoccupied with the welfare of the colonies and with Ben Franklin's mission to London.

The most serious problem faced by Nathaniel Greene was the conflict between his desire to join the Kentish Guards and his desire to maintain a good relationship with his Quaker Friends. Greene was certain that preparation for war and willingness to fight was the only recourse available to the colonies if political liberty was to be maintained, yet he still held fervently to the peaceful ideals of his Quaker family and friends. Already he had been scolded by the Quaker Meeting for his warlike remarks. If he went to arms for the colonies, he would be read out of the Meeting and shunned by his own family. Nathaniel Greene was relieved that Kitty was not a Quaker and would not feel the loss of a lifetime of associations.

Nathaniel and his cousin Griffin publicly announced their willingness to join battle against British suppression of American rights by attending a military rally and exhibition at Plainfield, Connecticut. Though their Quaker Meeting had no evidence that they had actually joined the Guards, notice was taken of the Greenes' improper interest in martial matters. A committee to investigate the activities of the two young men found their conduct inappropriate for Quakers. In June 1774 the clerk of the Meeting recorded that "as they had not given this Meeting any satisfaction for their misconduct, therefore this Meeting doth put them from under the care of the Meeting." Nathaniel was among the first of many young Quaker men torn by a conflict of moral codes. Though some chose to repudiate the call to arms, others felt compelled to forsake their beloved Quaker heritage.

Since Kitty was not a Quaker, her marriage to Nathaniel Greene served to estrange him further from the Friends. She was a young society woman and too frivolous and scandalously clothed for the tastes of many in the Quaker Meeting. Kitty had just turned eighteen when she became Nathaniel Greene's pretty bride on July 20, 1774. The newlyweds were brought closer by impending war and religious controversy. Kitty was soon pregnant and Nat began to dream of a large family to fill the house in Coventry and drown out the silence from his Quaker Friends. Their marriage, which began in William and Catherine Greene's mansion in East Greenwich, remained happy in spite of the lengthy separations and wartime privations that followed.

Upon hearing the news from Lexington, Massachusetts, on the night of the first pitched battle of the Revolutionary War in April 1775, the Kentish Guards assembled in Providence with Sam Ward at their head as colonel. A messenger from Governor Warton explained to them the military positions about Cambridge and Boston, but the expedition to the city was delayed a few days for organizational changes since the rebel positions were secure for the present.

The Rhode Island Assembly convened to fast and pray and to elect a committee for discussions with Connecticut on the common defense of New England. In his absence Samuel Ward, Jr. could not be appointed to the committee to serve as a delegate to the Continental Congress in Philadelphia, so Nathaniel Greene was chosen in his place.

The little-exercised Kentish Guards contributed their best to the Rhode Island forces, which numbered about 1,500. A commanding officer was needed for these eight companies, and Nathaniel Greene was chosen. Apparently, the more obvious two choices, the major general of the militia and Colonel Varnum of the Kentish Guards, declined the post. The choice by the assembly was fortunate, for they had obtained a man of integrity and wide exposure to the classics of military history. Nineteen-year-old Kitty Greene was as surprised as anyone that her husband had received the rank of brigadier general.

Before he could lead the Rhode Island forces to a Cambridge encampment, Nathaniel Greene felt constrained to assign responsibility for his private affairs to his brother. He sent an order to his tailor for a uniform to be delivered at Cambridge the next week. Just before he left Providence, Nat composed a letter to Kitty at Coventry:

> My dear wife—I am at this moment going to set off for camp, having been detained by the Committee of Safety till now. I have not so much in my mind that wounds my peace, as the separation from you. My bosom is knitted to yours by all the gentle feelings that inspire the softest sentiments of conjugal love. It had been happy for me if I could have lived a private life in peace and plenty, enjoying all the happiness that results from a well-tempered society founded on mutual esteem.

But the injury done my country and the chains of slavery forging for posterity, calls me forth to defend our common rights, and repel the bold invaders of the sons of freedom. I hope the righteous God that rules the world will bless the armies of America, and receive the spirits of those whose lot it is to fall in action into the paradise of God, and into whose protection I commend you and myself; and am, with truest regard, your loving husband, N. Greene.

Kitty was too young and too recently married to be content with the protection of God and her husband's brother, instead of the conjugal embrace of her husband.

When he reached the colonial camp at Cambridge, Nathaniel Greene found Artemas Ward to be the general of the Massachusetts forces. Each colony's forces were encamped as separate units with separate officer corps, paymasters, and commissaries. On June 15, 1775 George Washington was named commander in chief of the Continental armies, and his eight brigadiers included Greene of Rhode Island. The commander in chief arrived in Cambridge on July 2. The community at headquarters waxed quite friendly as General Washington grew comfortable in command of the Continentals. Greene wrote home to Kitty describing the atmosphere at camp:

I am now going to dine with his Excellency General Washington, I wish you could fly to Cambridge and partake of a friendly repast.

When Martha Washington arrived in Boston and the Commander made it clear that other officers' wives were welcome, Kitty Greene traveled to Boston in time for Christmas. She brought with her a son born since Nat had gone to war. While a baby George Washington Greene heard the guns of war in Boston. Kitty's exuberance endeared her to Martha Washington, and she became a welcome guest in the commander in chief's household. There was courage in these officers' wives who met at Christmas headquarters, since, in addition to fear for their husbands, the women themselves were in some danger. There were many severe shortages, especially of firewood. Some troops actually had no cooking fire and devoured raw and frozen meat. The siege of Boston ended with British withdrawal at the end of the winter just as the wives began to return to their homes.

When the situation outside New York seemed stabilized, the wives once again gathered in the countryside. Kitty stayed in Rhode

Island longer than most because she hesitated to leave her son with her husband's brother. Yet she also felt a summer in the diseased environment of an army camp would be unhealthy. Intimate and confidential messages flurried between Kitty and Nathaniel Greene. When Kitty finally headed for New York, the long-awaited British assault had begun and Nathaniel Greene was gravely ill with fever. Kitty was forced to turn back to Rhode Island, though she might have refused to do so had she known of her husband's condition.

During the next two years, Nathaniel Greene became George Washington's most reliable second in leadership. In 1777 Greene represented the commander in chief at Congress and acquitted himself well. Kitty was at the time confined in Rhode Island awaiting the birth of their second child and must have sometimes wondered what marvelous sights her husband was viewing in the glamorous wartime capital of Philadelphia. Shortly after Nat left Congress for Morristown headquarters, Kitty delivered a daughter, who was named Martha for Mrs. Washington. She was quite ill after this birth, and though Kitty suppressed that news in her own letters, the neighbors and his brother informed Nathaniel. He arranged for her to stay with a family of friends near the camp and told her that she could also learn music and French in the household. Nathaniel Greene's brief visit to Philadelphia had encouraged him to think of the cultural life which his wife might enjoy after the war. Life at Morristown was pleasant and the women continued amusements which were frugal but enjoyable—masks, games, concerts, dinners, and sewing circles. The wives scattered home once again with the first trumpets of resumed conflict late in the summer of 1777.

After the war all of those who had been there agreed that Kitty Greene's most memorable service to the cause had occurred in the winter encampment at Valley Forge in 1778. She had left her two infants with the family in Rhode Island in order to arrive at Valley Forge in late February. The journey was exhausting, but she felt healthier than just after her daughter's birth. Her energy did not flag at camp. With only a limited knowlege of French and her own natural enthusiasm, Kitty brought the European volunteers to her little cabin in droves. In the third week of February, the famine at camp was so severe that the situation seemed hopeless, and the soldiers were naked beyond not only comfort and health, but also modesty. To save the army, General Washington resorted to seizure of food, blankets, and forage. To manage the acquisition of resources, Washington assigned Nathaniel Greene to the post of quartermaster general of the army.

By sharing their husbands' privations and sympathizing with the soldiers' bitter lot, the wives at Valley Forge may have helped hold down desertions and keep the army together. Their diversions helped preserve sanity on the part of the distracted and almost despairing officer corps, and just their presence in such adverse conditions tipped the balance toward survival. On May 6 the survivors celebrated the completion of the French alliance by performing a difficult precision drill. Though mere skeletons, these men displayed pride in their training, in their uniforms mended by the ladies, and in their very survival. Kitty left camp and headed home to her two babies, accompanied by her quartermaster husband as far as the Hudson.

A few days after his return to camp, Nathaniel Greene resumed correspondence with his absent wife. As always in the field, Nathaniel strove in every letter to show hope for the future and to leave no important questions unanswered in case he failed to survive to write again. Though he was harried by his duties, he wrote:

> I have only time to tell you now that I am here in the usual style, writing, scolding, eating, and drinking, but there is no Mrs. Greene to spend an agreeable hour with. I hope you got safe home. [*sic*] Pray write me a full history of family matters; there is nothing will be so agreeable. Kiss the sweet little children for their absent papa. You must make yourself as happy as possible; write me if you are in want of anything to render you so.

Both Greenes knew that another child would be born before the summer's end.

The next winter when Kitty arrived at Middlebrook headquarters, she brought with her two little girl babies and four-year-old George. By bringing her children to camp, Kitty showed tremendous faith. She believed that the supply situation would not be as desperate as it had been at Valley Forge, partly because her husband was quartermaster general. The war had been going on for four years, and Kitty wanted desperately to experience something like a normal family life with her husband and children at the family board.

When the party season began after a happy winter, Kitty had recovered her health and figure from her third delivery. At a small party when she recklessly announced that she could dance forever, General Washington took up the challenge, and Greene seated himself with Mrs. Washington and kept careful track of the time. Later he wrote a friend in Rhode Island:

> We had a dance at my quarters a few evenings past. His Excellency and Mrs. Greene danced upwards of three hours without once sitting down. Upon the whole, we had a pretty little frisk.

The winter passed easily and quickly and departures from headquarters were made with deep regrets.

Next winter the family was once again reunited at the Middlebrook headquarters. Kitty Greene made a hazardous and almost ill-fated journey through the blizzards to reach camp only a short while before the birth of her fourth child, Nathaniel Ray Greene. The whole army rejoiced when the baby screamed its first breath in the chilled cottage. Kitty responded with tears when the soldiers brought little toys of precious wood carved by frozen fingers to the newborn and his mother. The sheer terror of such conditions for childbirth—a blizzard, freezing temperatures, and a revolutionary war winter camp—was impressive testimony to the personal courage of Kitty Greene.

When the southern front became important after the loss of Charleston and Gates's blundering, George Washington assigned Nathaniel Greene to that command. Greene was desirous of a lengthy home visit before journeying to such dangerous duty so far from his family, but the commander in chief refused the indulgence he had denied himself. Before receiving Washington's insistence on a rapid departure south, Greene had decided that the southern front was too critical to hazard a lapse in command. His real concern was that Kitty had already begun her trip to his winter encampment.

Once again Nathaniel Greene wrote his wife a letter which he knew would arouse a multitude of reasonable fears for his safety. He also knew that she would feel keen disappointment at having journeyed so far to no avail.

> My Dear Angel
> I am this moment setting off for the Southward, having kept expresses flying all night to see if I could hear anything of you. But as there was not the least intelligence of your being on the road, necessity obliges

me to depart. As I shall ride very fast, and make a stop on only one or two days at Headquarters and about the same time at Philadelphia, it will be impossible for you to catch up with me. Therefore, whatever things you have for me, you will please forward them by the express who will await you.

I have been almost distracted, I wanted to see you so much before I set out. My fears at being ordered southward was what made me hurry away Hubbard at such an early hour. God grant you patience and fortitude to bear the disappointment. My apprehensions for your safety distress me exceedingly. If heaven preserves us until we meet, our felicity will repay all the painful moments of a long separation. I am forever and forever yours, most sincerely and affectionately, NATH. GREENE.

Even as he left Philadelphia for the South, Nathaniel Greene had no news of his wife's travels. She had most probably despaired of getting to him in time and never left Coventry. During a year and a half of dangerous cat and mouse warfare in the swamps and fields of the Carolinas, the two Greenes would not be united.

The spring of 1782 offered a respite in the fighting and Nathaniel Greene sent for Kitty. She had begun the journey from Coventry at the end of the previous year but was detained by inclement weather in Philadelphia in December. Philadelphia society celebrated the wife of the Quaker general whose successes in the Carolinas daily filled their papers. Friends persuaded her to leave seven-year-old George to be educated by Dr. Witherspoon, the president of Princeton. She finally met her husband's party in early April.

The morale of the camp was raised by Kitty Greene's effervescent presence, and she also revitalized the ladies on the neighboring war-ravaged plantations. With her genius for stimulating others to their most brilliant social efforts, Kitty Greene transformed the neighborhood into something like its prewar ambience. Though the army was as hungry and unclothed as usual, Kitty's warm spontaneity brought the troops closer to their commander than before her arrival. All were concerned when her physical stamina and spirits began to flag in the fever season of midsummer. She finally went to one of the sea islands for fresh air and fresh fruit. In a letter to an aide, Nathaniel Greene described Kitty's reception in South Carolina:

The people are very friendly, and strive to render this country agreeable to her, but the fevers fill her with apprehensions. She is a very great favorite, even with the ladies, and has almost rivalled me where I least expected it; her flowing tongue and cheerful countenance quite triumph over my grave face. I bear it with great philosophy, as I gain on one hand what I lose on the other.

When Nathaniel was struck with fevers in September, Kitty rushed to his side from her island retreat, only to find him well enough to write Congress begging for food, clothes, and medical care for his weakened men.

When Charleston was finally evacuated by the British, supplies were so short that the planned celebration of its liberation had to be curtailed. Greene advertised for bids to supply his empty commissary and received only one, from a Banks who claimed to be a Virginian. Most army contractors were fraudulent to some degree, but Banks was a smooth talker who could deceive even the shrewd and experienced Greene. Perhaps compassion for his men led him to blindness if only they could be clothed and fed. Banks did help prevent complete degeneration of the army to starvation and nakedness; unfortunately, he also involved Greene's name in various other shady credit practices. From that time until Kitty's death years later, the Greenes were haunted by the necessity of doing the honorable thing and making good on Banks's transactions. There were just enough people jealous of Nathaniel Greene's reputation to fuel rumors that he had been fully aware of Banks's maneuvers.

On December 14, 1782, there was an evacuation ball in Charleston at which army minstrels played minuets together with the Virginia reel. Decorations were magnolia leaves, paper flowers, and bunting. There were few refreshments, but that failed to dampen Kitty Greene's enthusiasm for dancing with all the young officers under her husband's indulgent eye. Kitty made many conquests, but it was her husband whom she relied upon to come home when the war was over as he had promised years earlier. When she sailed for home on the first transport in July, she happily anticipated the realization of the dream which she had shared with Nathaniel since the war began so shortly after their marriage. She had a shopping spree in Philadelphia and then gathered her children whom she had not seen for more than a year. Predictably, when Kitty went home to Rhode Island, she was pregnant with her fifth child.

In gratitude for her services, the Georgia legislature granted to General Greene a sequestered Loyalist estate which included a very nice plantation on the Savannah River called Mulberry Grove.

Greene finally moved his family to Georgia in the fall of 1785. At forty-three, Nathaniel began work to restore the neglected grounds. Meanwhile, he searched desperately for means and time to make good on the Banks debts for which he had probably not been responsible. Nine months after the family moved south, Kitty Greene was a widow with five small children and a debt-ridden estate. The nation had needed her husband in the revolutionary war era, but when the conflict was over, it did not provide for the security of Catherine or her children.

After her husband's death Catherine Greene relied upon the children's tutor, Phineas Miller, for the management of the estate. Miller was a Yale University graduate who was deeply impressed with the general's glamorous wife. Mulberry Grove became a gathering place for the cultured of Georgia in the winters, and Kitty visited her family in Newport in the summer season each year.

On her return from Newport in 1792, Eli Whitney became a traveling companion and then a houseguest. Observing his ingenuity in the design of a new tambour frame, Kitty Greene suggested he apply his talents to the problem of stripping seeds from short-staple cotton to make it profitable. Whitney worked behind closed doors in a basement room for six months and completed a model of an engine for the purpose. When Kitty called in her neighbors to view Whitney's invention, she accomplished a revolution in southern agriculture. Phineas Miller and Eli Whitney set up a corporation and applied for a patent, but litigation costs and the simplicity of the machine itself prevented them from ever gaining from the invention. In 1795 Catherine Greene committed her entire estate to the protection of the patent. She married Phineas Miller in 1796 and lost Mulberry Grove in 1800. Phineas Miller died in 1803, Eli Whitney died in 1807, and Catherine Greene Miller died of a fever in 1814 at the age of fifty-nine.

18

Abigail Adams

SEPTEMBER 1777 in Braintree, Massachusetts. In the clear fall light, the quiet town—ten miles from the noise and crowds of Boston—seemed far from the war. In the spacious kitchen of a farmhouse, Abigail Adams sat alone before her table, holding an envelope she had just received.

Her hand shook with fear, and she put the letter down, unable to open it. It was from Philadelphia where John was with the Continental Congress, but it was not an eagerly-awaited message from her husband. Rather, it carried the frank of James Lovell, a friend of John's and a fellow delegate from Massachusetts. Abigail was terror-stricken, for a letter with his colleague's frank could only mean that John was unable to write himself—that he was captured, ill, or dead.

Abigail had already suffered much from John's involvement in politics. It had begun with his defense of the British troops who were arrested after the Boston Massacre in 1770, long before the outbreak of the Revolution.

Eight soldiers and their captain, Thomas Preston, were charged with murder after the incident. Patriot feeling in Boston was so intense that no lawyer would risk the anger of the mob by taking the defense of the troops.

But Adams took the case. It brought him into conflict with his cousin Samuel Adams, who, along with his friends John Hancock, James Warren, and James Otis, had for months been inciting the less stable elements of Boston against the British. Their agitation had led to the irresponsible harassment of the British that resulted in the shootings. For Adams the case was crucial; a fair trial and a competent defense would prove to the crown and the other

256

colonists that law and justice, rather than mob anarchy, prevailed in Boston.

Adams was joined in the defense by Josiah Quincy, who had agreed to take the case only if Adams would work with him. They delayed the trial for over six months to give public feeling time to cool down, and prepared a careful defense.

At the trial Adams relentlessly cross-examined the witnesses until the truth emerged. It had been no peaceful gathering of citizens deliberately fired upon by belligerent redcoats, but a mob of troublemakers—"a motley rabble of saucy boys, Negroes, and mulattoes, Irish teagues and outlandish jack tars," he called them. They had taunted the soldiers until, frightened beyond endurance, one soldier and then the others fired, killing three persons in the mob.

Preston was released after a hearing determined that he had not given an order to fire, and all but two of the soldiers were acquitted. The two were convicted of manslaughter and released after having their thumbs branded and reading from the Bible.

For Adams it was a victory not only of law over mob rule, but also an assertion of his political independence from the pressure of popular feeling. It was a victory too over the harassment he withstood during the trial. His home was damaged, rocks were thrown through his windows, and he was insulted on the street. The harassment only made him all the more determined to stand his ground, and through it all Abigail stood with him. Even after the trial, the attacks continued. Since they had lost the case in court, the more hotheaded and unthinking Patriots attacked Adams through the columns of Boston's newspapers.

However, Adams's integrity won him greater popularity with the more serious Patriot leaders in Boston, and in the spring of 1770 they elected him delegate to the General Court from the town of Boston. Adams accepted the post with a sense of martyrdom; he was throwing away a promising, even brilliant, career as lawyer for a political cause that would do him little good. His sole motive for getting involved was his sense of duty to the country.

When Abigail heard the news of John's election, she burst into tears. She was pregnant with Charles, her third child, and she wanted a stable family life. But she decided it was important that the best men take leadership in the colonies for the good of the country. This was only the first time that she would give up John for this reason.

John's involvement in the politics of independence deepened with each new incident. After the Boston Tea Party, he was elected to the First Continental Congress that convened in September 1774. He was also a member of the Second Continental Congress that drafted the Declaration of Independence, and he signed it. He knew that his signature would hang him if the British ever got hold of him.

John was away in Philadelphia in 1776 while Abigail, in Braintree, had the war at her doorstep. Washington had moved his forces to take possession of Boston in the spring, and from her home Abigail watched the battles and lay awake nights listening to the roaring of cannon. "I have been kept in a continual state of anxiety and expectation ever since you left me," she wrote to John then. "But hark! The house this instant shakes with the roar of cannon . . . no sleep for me tonight." And a day or two later: "I could no more sleep than if I had been in the engagement; the rattling of the windows, the jar of the house, the continual roar of twenty-four pounders, and the bursting of shells, give us such ideas, and realize a scene to us of which we could form scarcely any conception. . . . To-night we shall realize a more terrible scene still." This time it turned out well; Washington took the hills around Boston, and the British decided to leave the town.

From near her home, Abigail watched an unfolding panorama of one of the largest military movements of the war. "From Penn's Hill we have a view of the largest fleet ever seen in America," she wrote, awed by the sight. "You may count upwards of a hundred and seventy sail. They look like a forest."

In the fall of 1777 there was no such impressive sight of British defeat, nor such a clear view of the tide of battle. The year had seen a great deal of military action, but nothing had been decisive. In January Washington had won a bold victory at Princeton, and the frustrated Howe had taken his army back to New York City where he idled. Meanwhile the Americans and the other British forces spent the spring trying to get in position to deal each other a solid defeat.

John had left early in January, and Abigail stayed to follow the course of the war and worry by herself. Battles were being fought all over New York State, and she asked John to get her a map of the northern states so that she could follow the actions in the field.

Now in the middle of September, she still had not received the map from him. There had been many reversals for the American forces; rumors ran wild in the air; and she had a letter from her husband's friend instead of from John himself. Her mind was inflamed with fears; she wrote later of ˙

> the agitation and distress I was thrown into by receiving a letter in his handwriting, franked by him. It seems almost impossible that the human mind could take in, in so small a space of time, so many ideas as rushed upon mine in the space of a moment. I cannot describe to you what I felt. The sickness or death of the dearest of friends, with ten thousand horrors, seized my imagination. I took up the letter, then laid it down, then gave it out of my hand unable to open it, then collected resolution enough to unseal it but dared not read it; began at the bottom—read a line—then attempted to begin it, but could not.

"I pray heaven," she concluded, "I may never realize such another moment of distress," and closed her letter with words of joy and gratitude that John was alive: "Good night, friend of my heart, companion of my youth, husband, and lover. Angels watch thy repose!"

Enough had happened for Abigail's fears to be real. All summer the British had been following a plan to crush the rebellion in the northern states. And in July Burgoyne took Fort Ticonderoga, on the south point of Lake Champlain. Its defenders evacuated the fort rather than attempting to hold it against the attackers. Abigail was shocked and outraged. When she wrote John about the news, she accused the Americans of cowardice and treachery, of bringing dishonor on the new nation. She raged at "the disgrace brought upon our arms," and hoped that "the inquiry will be made," and that "if cowardice, guilt, deceit, are found upon any one, howsoever high or exalted his station, may shame, reproach, infamy, hatred, and the execrations of the public be his portion."

"It is to be lamented," she wrote, "that we have not men among ourselves sufficiently qualified for war to take upon them the most important command."

Abigail's anger was misdirected for she did not know that the evacuation had been a wise tactical decision. Burgoyne had attacked with 8,000 redcoats, Canadian troops, and Indians. In the face of this overwhelming force, the Americans did not panic, but rather made an orderly retreat to Fort Edward, forty-five miles to the south on the Hudson.

To Abigail, far from the fighting, it looked like the war was being lost. And there were other things that fed her anxiety. In Boston food and other necessities were scarce, and fear wracked the city. She had complained to John earlier that "the merchant scolds, the farmer growls, and every one seems wroth that he cannot grind his neighbor." After Ticonderoga she saw the scolding give way to hoarding and gouging, and then to riot. She told John of a coffee merchant who, having a large stock of coffee that he refused to sell for less than twice the going price, was attacked by a mob of women. They threw him into a cart and hauled him off to his warehouse, and when he still refused to hand over the keys, they beat him until he finally gave in. Once they had the keys, the mob turned its attention to the warehouse, and the merchant escaped while the women hauled away the coffee. A large crowd of men watched the battle, Abigail noted, "amazed, silent spectators of the whole transaction."

The only thing unusual about the riot was that the attackers were all women. John made light of it, writing to Abigail that "you have made me merry with the female frolic with the miser," but he did not have to see it every day. Abigail lived in the midst of the turmoil, and she saw the city falling apart as store after store was broken into by mobs, and the coffee, sugar, and other goods were carried off.

She stood apart from the riots and attacks on merchants, preferring to go without rather than join a mob, but she was not immune to the fear that gripped her neighbors. The day after the women's coffee riot, the British fleet was sighted off Cape Ann, just thirty-five miles up the coast from Boston. Fear of invasion gripped the city, and panic spread. Abigail herself made plans to leave, and she saw the last remainders of community spirit crumble in the panic to escape:

> All Boston was in confusion packing up and carting out of town household furniture, military stores, goods, etc. Not less than a thousand teams were employed on Friday and Saturday; and to their shame be it told, not a small trunk would they carry under eight dollars, and many of them, I am told, asked a hundred dollars a load; for carting a hogshead of molasses eight miles, thirty dollars. O human nature! or rather, O inhuman nature! what art thou? . . . though pretty weak, I set about packing my things, and on Saturday removed a load.

The invasion did not come after all—for Howe was merely sailing

in circles trying to decide what to do about Philadelphia—and
Abigail stayed in Braintree.

Abigail's steadfastness in the midst of war's turmoil led John to
think about the support wives gave to leaders of nations. In subtle
appreciation, he told Abigail that great men would not be so were it
not for the women who helped them. "Upon examining the
biography of illustrious men," he told Abigail, "you will generally
find some female about them, in the relation of mother or wife or
sister" who encouraged them. John even went so far as to blame the
behavior of the British commanders on their spouses. General
Howe and his brother, admiral of the fleet in America, had been
sailing off the coast for weeks; the troops and horses suffered on the
airless and confining ships. Everyone was baffled by this behavior,
and John concluded that

> . . . the Howes cannot have very great women for wives. If they had,
> we should suffer more from their exertions than we do . . . A woman
> of good sense would not let her husband spend five weeks at sea in
> such a season of the year. A smart wife would have put Howe in
> possession of Philadelphia a long time ago.

Howe's immediate actions did not make much sense, but he was
not quite the fool John presented to Abigail. He eventually landed
his troops at the northernmost point of Chesapeake Bay and set off
toward Philadelphia. When John learned of this, he must have been
alarmed, for he bolstered his spirits with an incredibly optimistic
view of the situation.

He poured out confidence to Abigail. At the end of August, he
pompously told her that "Howe will make but a pitiful figure. . . .
The Continental Army . . . is in my opinion more numerous by
several thousands than Howe's whole force. I am afraid that he will
be frightened, and run on board his ships, and go away plundering
to some other place." John was even convinced that the Americans
looked too formidable for their own good!

In the meantime prices were raging in Philadelphia, and along
with detailed speculations on Washington's strategy, John faithfully
reported "prices current" in his letters to Abigail. Most of his
thoughts, though, were on the strategy of the two commanders and
the outcome.

On September 8 he told Abigail of "a very general apprehension"
in Philadelphia; the two huge armies were near the city, but there

had been no engagement yet; John was anxiously distressed. Three days later the suspense was relieved: Howe defeated Washington at Brandywine. The battle was only thirty miles from the city, and Washington lost a thousand men—nearly a tenth of his forces.

In another week Howe was at Chester, just fifteen miles away, and John's confidence began to evaporate as reality intruded. Abigail found his thoughts turning to the escape of Congress and the silver lining in the clouds:

> How much longer Congress will stay is uncertain. I hope we shall not remove until the last necessity, that is, until it shall be rendered certain that Mr. Howe will get the city . . . don't be anxious about me, nor about our great and sacred cause. It is the cause of truth and will prevail.

With Howe getting ever closer to her husband, Abigail received the letter that struck such terror in her heart. She finally summoned the courage to open it and accept its news, whatever it might be. She was suddenly relieved: the letter assured her of John's health and contained the map of the states she had wanted. John had asked Lovell—his good friend, fellow citizen of Boston, and colleague—to find one for him.

To Lovell it seemed a perfect opportunity, since his interest in Abigail had gone beyond affection for the wife of a friend. He got the map, and instead of giving it to John he sent it to Abigail himself, and along with it a letter intimating his feelings for her. "I could not with delicacy have told him to his face that your having given your heart to such a man is what, most of all, makes me yours," he wrote. If she read the passage one way, it was simply a declaration of his admiration for John, but she couldn't help seeing also that Lovell was telling her of his admiration for her.

When Abigail told John about getting the map, she mentioned only that Lovell had "accompanied it with a very polite letter." Lovell's declaration was, she thought, peculiar, but it aroused her interest.

The fears she had experienced upon receipt of the letter had just cause considering the events of the war. In the early morning of September 19, the British had taken a ford on the Schuylkill River, just a few miles west of Philadelphia and only a day's march from the city. The papers of Congress were hurriedly packed and sent to Bristol, a town on the Delaware several miles east of Philadelphia. The members of Congress packed their belongings and fled to York

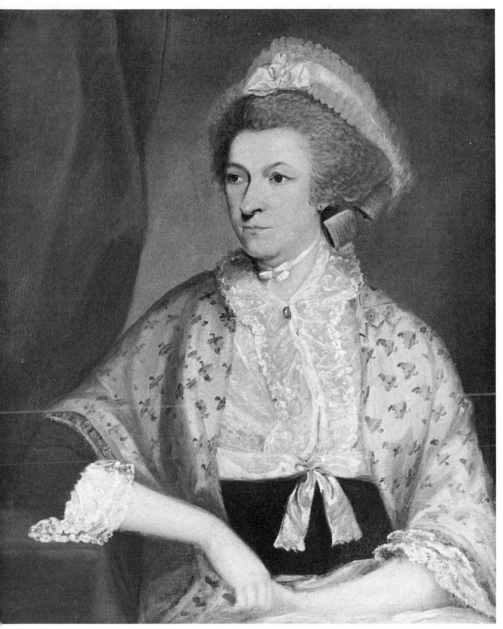

Abigail Adams (Portrait by Ralph Earl)
Courtesy, New York State Historical Association, Cooperstown

ninety miles to the west, which now became the capital. A week later, Howe occupied Philadelphia and settled down for a comfortable winter in the most cosmopolitan and sophisticated of the new nation's cities.

With the fall of Philadelphia, Abigail was suddenly in the dark about what was happening in that part of the country. She had heard rumors about Washington's defeats at Brandywine and Germantown and more rumors about Congress fleeing Philadelphia, but she had no hard news and no letters from John. Nor could she send a message to him. The lack of news could mean that John was ill or dead; it could mean that the British had taken the capital; or it could simply mean that the mail service was a little more erratic than usual. She could not tell which of these was the more likely possibility.

She wrote to John early in October, sending the letter by a friend who promised to find John wherever he was and give him the letter personally. She filled it with bits and pieces of rumored military actions, the anxious hope that Howe would not get Philadelphia, and resignation to fate: "Tis a day of doubtful expectations. Heaven only knows our destiny."

She did not know as she wrote that Howe had been in Philadelphia for two weeks.

Her next letter from John brought her happy news. He was in York, safe from the British, living with friends in a comfortable house. His health was good but he was worn down with the cares of office, he explained, and he longed "with the utmost impatience to come home." With the loss of the capital and Washington's debacle at Germantown, his mood was gloomy. Abigail, too, was upset by the loss of the capital—"If men will not fight and defend their own particular spot, if they will not drive the enemy from their doors, then they deserve the subjection which awaits them," she declared to him.

She had to resort to grabbing at straws to sustain her morale: "Providence for wise purpose has oftentimes since the commencement of this war brought about our deliverance by ways and means which have appeared to us the most improbable and unlikely."

Abigail had good news from the north the next week. Burgoyne was getting deeper in the mire. She could not know it then, but the Americans were at the turning point of the war.

After he took Ticonderoga, Burgoyne followed the Americans to Fort Edward in order to demolish them there. But the terrain was rough, and with all the dependents to protect and feed and all their baggage to haul, it took him nearly a month to get to Fort Edward.

When he got there, the fort had already been evacuated. Burgoyne thought the Americans were on the run. The Patriots in fact were in some trouble—morale was low, discipline poor, and disorder rampant—but it was not due to Burgoyne. It was due rather to Congress, which was wrangling over the choice of a commander for the northern army. Finally the command went to Horatio Gates, a man whose main talent was for getting on well with politicians. Gates was disliked by his fellow officers; he was careful to stay out of danger in battle; he had little character or ideas of his own; and he was incompetent.

While the question of command was being settled, the Americans retreated further south from Fort Edward, and Burgoyne sat waiting for supplies from Canada. By this time his lines of communication were impossibly overextended. His force was large, and he had many dependents. So he sent 700 men to Vermont to forage. They were supposed to cover a large area and return in a few days with grain, cattle, horses, and whatever other useful things they found. The Green Mountain boys got them all before they even crossed the Vermont border. A second party of 300 men was lost in the same way; Burgoyne had spent fully an eighth of his force simply trying to feed the rest.

Burgoyne was as yet only a little worried, and still hoping to find food and supplies, he crossed to the west bank of the Hudson and headed south. Now he began to realize just how much trouble he was in, for the harassment from local Patriots was so intense that he could advance barely a mile a day.

The armies battled each other on September 12 at Freeman's Farm. Gates nearly lost out of sheer stupidity, and the victory came only because Benedict Arnold turned back Burgoyne with a small force.

Burgoyne's situation steadily worsened. The militia cut his lines of communication with Canada completely, so he could no longer retreat. On October 7 he made a last ditch attempt to break out of his trap. Arnold again saved the day. Ten days later, after a discussion of terms, Burgoyne surrendered. Gates took all the credit for this, and some people in Congress began talking about giving him Washington's command. Arnold received no thanks.

Abigail was ecstatic. To her, Burgoyne's surrender seemed the fulfillment of her earlier hopes; it seemed even divinely ordained. In celebration she took a ride to town with her daughter Nabby, "to join . . . with my friends in thanksgiving and praise to the Supreme Being who hath so remarkably delivered our enemies into our hands." It gave her real consolation, for the war and John's political service caused her hardship. At the time of Burgoyne's surrender, she and John had been married for thirteen years, and they had been "cruelly separated" for the last three. But the brighter horizons that now beckoned the new country made this seem worthwhile:

> I have, patiently as I could, endured it, with the belief that you were serving your country and rendering your fellow-creatures essential benefits. May future generations rise up and call you blessed, and the present behave worthy of the blessings you are laboring to secure to them, and I shall have less reason to regret the deprivation of my own particular felicity. Adieu, dearest of friends, adieu.

Abigail's happiness was not just a matter of being with her husband; she was gratified by John's stature as a national leader and his work in building the new country. And she was the woman behind the nation-builder, a woman like those John had talked of finding in the biographies of "illustrious men."

Abigail was even happy at the extremely easy surrender terms Gates had given. "Many people find fault with them," she wrote, "but perhaps do not consider sufficiently the circumstances of General Gates, who, by delaying and exacting more, might have lost all . . . he has followed the Golden Rule, and done as he would wish himself, in like circumstances, to be dealt with." This was perhaps Gates's motive, but Abigail did not know that his terms had been inappropriately generous, nor did she know of his incompetence and his fraud in taking credit for the surrender.

John, for his part, was happy that it was Gates to whom Burgoyne surrendered, for had it been Washington, "idolatry and adulation would have been unbounded; so excessive as to endanger our liberties . . . now we can allow a certain citizen to be wise, virtuous, and good, without thinking him a deity or a savior."

Ironically, the events of the war would show Washington to be a savior, and he would receive the idolatry that John feared.

In November John was at last about to start on his long and cold journey home as Congress adjourned. Abigail, who had been longing for him, sent him a coyly understated promise of the welcome she had in mind: "Let the thought of the cordial reception you will be assured of meeting warm the cold wintry blasts and make your return joyful. Adieu."

Abigail had John to herself for only a short time. He arrived at the turn of the year, and in the middle of February he returned to his duties, leaving her alone to manage the farm, raise the family, and soothe her pain at his departure.

John was then appointed commissioner to France. He and Abigail agonized over whether or not he should accept the post. John was torn between duty to his country—and the honor and excitement of the new post—and his desire to be with Abigail. She was torn between her desire to keep him with her and her wish to see him a great man of his country. She decided that she could find happiness in seeing John follow the call of his nation, and for his part he decided to take on the burdens of this most major step in establishing the new country's foreign relations.

This time the parting was much harder for Abigail. John took their ten-year-old son, John Quincy, with him. He was not going to Philadelphia, nor even a hundred miles farther to York, but all the way to Paris.

In France John had the difficult task of becoming accustomed to a foreign culture. He knew little French and less of French ways. He was amazed by the magnificence of Paris and scandalized by French morals and luxury. He had difficult affairs to conduct, and the Americans in Paris, who should have been helpful, were instead split by conniving factions that schemed against each other. He had to straighten out the affairs of his predecessor, Silas Deane.

While John moved through the exciting, glittering world of Paris, Abigail carried on as best she could in Braintree. She was very lonely without John and her son and felt even more isolated from them since mail service across the Atlantic was so poor. But at least she had with her Nabby—who at thirteen was beginning to turn into a woman—and young Charles, her favorite.

To keep her spirits up, Abigail carried on a flirtation with her cousin John Thaxter, who was John's law clerk. Thaxter, who was unmarried and without a lover, visited often and listened entranced as Abigail titillated him—and herself—with long, rapturous descriptions of the pleasures of marriage. When he too went away to Philadelphia, she wrote him, "I feel very lonely and miss you exceedingly."

Fortunately, she still had Lovell to give her at least some solace in her loneliness. Before John left, Lovell had asked him to intercede with Abigail on his behalf. He had written her too fervent a letter, and she had scolded him and withdrawn.

But now she was ready for a reconciliation. She was facing a long absence from John, and even the voyage itself gave her cause to worry. And so she replied to Lovell through Thaxter. He had been partly responsible for John's leaving, she told him, so he had the responsibility of keeping her informed of what was going on in the capital. Her interest in politics was of course genuine, but Lovell made a more than convenient correspondent to keep her up to date on the affairs of Congress.

Lovell took her explicit invitation as a green light. First he wrote protesting his innocence of any offense to her, telling her that his sentiments were those of admiration for his friend's wife for whom he wished nothing more than happiness with her husband. Having established his own disguise, he took every chance to write more boldly. Abigail maintained her masquerade of shock at Lovell's insinuations and declarations. As he used his mantle of innocence to phrase subtle expressions of desire, so she used the pose of the shocked Puritan to invite and enjoy them.

She scolded him for writing her letters without formal salutations, for his was an intimate form. He replied, "Must I only write to you in the language of gazettes? Must I suppress opinion, sentiment, and just encomium upon the gracefulness of a lovely suffering wife or mother?" He was saddened by her rejection of his sentiments, and so now he would keep his feelings to himself and forgive her for "calling names and misconstruing the honest sentiments of your sincere servant." In all events, they continued their double-edged correspondence.

Abigail's communications with her husband were more dear to her but less possible. Though John wrote often, she seldom received his letters, and she had difficulty in finding a ship to take her letters to him. Ships were not scheduled; they each might hear of one leaving—with a captain who was willing to carry mail—only hours before it left. Abigail would hurriedly write a letter and then find someone to take it to the ship in Boston for her.

The voyage itself took four to six weeks. There was no assurance that the captain would care for the mail. There was the danger of British warships; captured letters might be printed in the English newspapers; and sometimes letters found their way into the American newspapers before they reached their addressees.

At the beginning of June, five months after he had left, John wrote to Abigail complaining "I have not received a line nor heard a word, directly or indirectly, concerning you, since my departure." He knew that the fault was the difficulty of the mail service, and he missed her deeply. He was enjoying France—"'Tis one great garden. Nature and art have conspired to render everything here delightful." But he was lonely for Abigail.

At the end of the month, he had at last "the inexpressible pleasure" of receiving a letter which Abigail had sent almost three months earlier. In the same month, Abigail, too, finally received one of John's letters—the first word from him in over five months. Up to then, she'd had only two bits of information of him: a mention, in a captured English newspaper, of his arrival in Paris; and a message from a ship captain.

Abigail wrote John of "the tears of joy" that filled her eyes when she saw his letter, of "the life of fear and anxiety" she had been leading since he had left her, of her happiness and gratitude that he was safe. She spoke too of her anger at the treatment of women in America, when compared with that of French women whom John had met. "I regret the trifling, narrow, contracted education of the females of my own country," she wrote. "You need not be told how much female education is neglected, nor how fashionable it has been to ridicule female learning." She would come to this theme again and again in her letters.

Abigail had other worries as well. There was tremendous inflation during the war and many necessities were difficult to get at any price. Since most clothing and manufactured goods were formerly imported from England, they were naturally scarce, and very expensive when they could be found. Also, with the large number of men in the militia, labor was scarce and expensive—Abigail worried about how she could possibly keep the farm going. John helped her somewhat by sending things from France—dresses, cloth, paper— but he could not help her with the day-to-day worries of running the farm. Her anxiety under such tight circumstances increased. The irregular mail from John irritated her, as did his reticence in the letters she received. She complained to him of "the very few lines I have received from you," and of his stiffness:

> I cannot take my pen, with my heart overflowing, and not give utterance to some of the abundance which is in it. Could you, after a thousand fears and anxieties, long expectation, and painful suspense, be satisfied with my telling you that I was well, that I wished you were

with me, that my daughter sent her duty, that I had ordered some articles for you, which I hoped would arrive, etc. etc? By Heaven, if you could, you have changed hearts with some frozen Laplander, or made a voyage to a region that has chilled every drop of your blood; but I will restrain a pen already, I fear, too rash, nor shall it tell you how much I have suffered from this appearance of—inattention.

When John read this he exploded:

For God's sake never reproach me again with not writing or with writing scraps. Your wounds are too deep. You know not, you feel not the dangers that surround me nor those that may be brought upon our country. Millions would not tempt me to write as I used. I have no security that every letter I write you will not be broken open, and copied, and transmitted to Congress and to English newspapers. They would find no treason nor deceit in them, it is true, but they would find weakness and indiscretion, which they would make as ill a use of.

He went on to detail his situation and to scold her for not understanding:

There are spies upon every word I utter, and every syllable I write. . . . My life has been often in danger, but I never considered my reputation and character so much in danger as now. I can pass for a fool, but I will not pass for a dishonest or mercenary man. Be on your guard, therefore. I must be on mine, and I will.

John was not exaggerating. Congress had taken away his commission so that he was now a private citizen in Paris, and he worried that some political enemy had made false accusations of him to Congress. He made ready to take a ship home whenever he could get one, and in the meantime he enjoyed himself traveling about.

Abigail was penitent after the blast she received from John; she replied lovingly that "the watery world alone can boast of large packets received . . . yet I will not be discouraged. I will persist in writing, though but one in ten should reach you."

John himself relented his scolding immediately after he had sent off his lecture to her. Abigail read in his next letter a conciliatory apology. Abigail was still lonesome for him, but after this exchange of feelings, she at least felt reassured.

It made it a bit easier for her to handle the problems she was having supporting the farm and taking care of the family. John's salary was barely adequate, and it was all he could do to support himself in Paris. He could not send money to Abigail, and Congress did not give her an allotment in consideration of having taken her husband away for the country's business.

Prices continued to soar in Boston. As the economic situation worsened, Abigail began having difficulty feeding her family. In three months molasses had risen from an expensive $12 a gallon to $20 a gallon; corn had gone from $25 a bushel to $80 a bushel. Meat was almost out of reach; board had long since become so expensive that Abigail had given up trying to keep her children at school. The money issued by the Continental Congress depreciated rapidly as soon as it came into circulation. Everyone preferred English money, but it was as scarce as English goods. "In contemplation of my situation," she wrote to John, "I am sometimes thrown into an agony of distress. Distance, dangers, and oh, I cannot name all the fears which sometimes oppress me, and harrow up my soul." Still, she found comfort in her faith that all would sooner or later be well: "Yet must the common lot of man one day take place . . . That we rest under the shadow of the Almighty is the consolation to which I resort, and find that comfort which the world cannot give."

Soon the situation was better, for John had found a ship and in August 1779 he came back to her. He brought their son with him; John Quincy was now a cultured young man.

Abigail and John had been separated for eighteen long months— difficult but fascinating months for John, difficult and wearing months for Abigail. Even now, John and Abigail's time together was pressed by the demands of others who wished to see him, and not the least of these demands were those of the country. John had been home only a short time when the state of Massachusetts called on him for help in creating its new constitution. It was hard work and it took John away from Abigail again, but at least he was in the state and not in Pennsylvania or Paris.

John was worried about his name in Congress. Partisans of other factions had made charges against him for his performance as commissioner in Paris. But Congress once again expressed its confidence in John by appointing him minister to negotiate peace with England. John would have to go to Paris again. He first declined the appointment, but his friends persuaded him to accept it.

He and Abigail discussed whether she and the children could go with him to Paris. They soon concluded that she could not leave; there was no one else to run the farm and not enough time to find a manager and arrange the countless details that would have to be taken care of. Moreover, John could not afford to keep the whole family in expensive Paris on his salary from Congress. They could not afford to board the children even in America, and Abigail would have to stay for this if for no other reason.

This time John's leaving was even harder on Abigail than his first departure for Paris, for he took not only John Quincy but Charles, her favorite child. He also took, as his private secretary, John Thaxter, Abigail's close friend, correspondent, and confidant.

They left in the middle of November. John had been home less than four months, and Abigail would not see him again for nearly five years.

As John left Braintree for Boston, Abigail faced her house, with only Nabby and seven-year old Tommy for company, and wrote to him.

> Dearest of Friends,
> My habitation, how disconsolate it looks! My table, I sit down to it, but cannot swallow my food! Oh, why was I born with so much sensibility, and why, possessing it, have I so often been called to struggle with it? I wish to see you again. Were I sure you would not be gone, I could not withstand the temptation of coming to town, though my heart would suffer over again the cruel torture of separation.

Her despondency was understandable. She had the farm to run and two children to raise, and not only was John gone but he had taken Thaxter with him.

Lovell did his best to keep her spirits up. He resumed his letter writing, keeping her informed of developments in Congress and sparking her amorous sensibilities. "How *do* you do, lovely Portia, these very cold days?" he wrote, calling her by her husband's favorite name for her, and adding suggestively, "Mistake me not willfully; I said days." In another letter he complained of the cold and the loneliness in his rooms and mentioned Ecclesiastes 4:11— but he did not write the words of the verse. Abigail was torn between her shock at the letter and her intense curiosity about what he was alluding to. When she finally gave in to her curiosity, she opened her Bible and read: "Again, if two lie together, then they have heat;

but how can one be warm alone?" Abigail was shocked—he was even using the Bible to stir her thoughts!

She was, of course, also pleased and excited. She wrote back scolding him as a "wicked man," but found a way, under the guise of talking on another subject, to return his attention. She felt that his words were a mocking imitation of *Tristram Shandy*, a novel which they had talked about in earlier letters. She had not read it because it was too frank about sex. Now she turned this discussion of literature into a witty and subtle appreciation of Lovell. Sterne's sexuality, she told Lovell, was "intermixed with a rich stream of benevolence flowing like milk and honey." He had, she continued, "an exquisite sensibility, a universal philanthropy—what a perverse genius he must have to hazard those fine powers and talents for a wicked wit." She went on to add a cautious excuse for her enjoyment of Lovell's words with a mock scolding: "I have charity enough for the writer to believe that his associates have been wholly of his own sex for three years past, or he could not have so offended."

Their affair by mail continued, and Lovell's admiration provided a romance and affection that sustained her while she coped with the day-to-day problems that grew increasingly serious. Inflation continued its upward spiral; by October 1880, prices were more than double what they had been eighteen months earlier. Yet despite the high price of labor, of food, of cloth, and of schooling, Abigail had managed always to keep the farm going, educate the children, and keep the family well-fed and clothed. Now she had only Nabby and Tommy to care for besides herself. She managed so well that she was able to add some more land—seven acres at the foot of Penn's hill—to the farm and even buy some land in Vermont that John had been interested in. With the farm running well, Abigail began to think of joining her husband in Europe.

She was anxious to see him, for she felt time catching up with them. In the late fall of 1782 after three years apart, she wrote to him, "Could we live to the age of the antediluvians, we might better support this separation; but, when threescore years and ten circumscribe the life of man, how painful is the idea that, of that short space, only a few years of social happiness are our allotted portion." But the passage was still too difficult to manage, and John was still too busy.

The war was lurching to a close. After the surrender of Burgoyne, the British had shifted their efforts to the southern states, but there too they had a rough time of it. Hoping for greater success farther north, Cornwallis had taken his army to Virginia, where at the Battle of Yorktown on October 18, 1781, he too surrendered. There was only small-scale fighting throughout the rest of the year and during 1782. With Yorktown the war was essentially over; the Americans had won, and the new country that Abigail's husband had worked for, and which had been her dream, was established. After a preliminary treaty was signed in late 1782, the final peace that John had labored for—the Treaty of Paris—was signed on February 3, 1783.

John was tired of the endless negotiations, the intrigue, and the diplomatic maneuvering. He had lost friends, some by treachery, some by honest disagreement; and he wanted to come home to Braintree and, most of all, to Abigail.

But Abigail and John both heard that he might be appointed to represent the new country as ambassador to Britain. And Abigail decided that she had had enough of their separation. She had not seen him and had barely heard from him for over four years. She had often written John of her desire to come to Europe, but it had never been possible. She felt more acutely than ever that she was wasting her life, separated from the man she loved. John too wanted to have Abigail with him in Europe, now that the arduous treaty negotiations were over and some stability could return to his life.

There were many problems. The affairs of the farm had to be settled, and someone had to be found to care for it.

But finally in June 1784, Abigail and her children left Boston on the merchant ship *Active*. They landed in England on July 20 after a difficult crossing. They found old friends in London, but Adams himself was in the Hague negotiating commercial treaties. On August 7, 1784 Abigail and John met for the first time in nearly five years. Their last separation was over.

Bibliography

ABIGAIL ADAMS

Adams, Charles Francis, ed. *Familiar Letters of John Adams and His Wife Abigail Adams, During the Revolution.* New York: The Riverside Press, 1875.

Adams, James Truslow. *The Adams Family.* New York: The Literary Guild, 1930.

Bobbe, Dorothie. *Abigail Adams, The Second First Lady.* New York: Minton, Balch, and Co., 1929.

Bradford, Gamaliel. *Portraits of American Women.* Boston: Houghton Mifflin Co., 1919.

Butterfield, Lyman H., ed. *The Adams Family Correspondence, December 1761-March 1778.* 2 vols. Cambridge: The Belknap Press of the Harvard University Press, 1963.

Minnigerode, Meade. *Some American Ladies: Seven Informal Biographies.* New York: G.P. Putnam's Sons, 1926.

Mitchell, Stewart, ed. *New Letters of Abigail Adams.* Boston: Houghton Mifflin Co., 1947.

Oliver, Andrew. *Portraits of John and Abigail Adams.* Cambridge: The Belknap Press of the Harvard University Press, 1967.

Richards, Laura E. *Abigail Adams and Her Times.* New York: D. Appleton and Co., 1917.

Smith, Page. *John Adams.* 2 vols. Garden City, N.Y.: Doubleday & Co., Inc., 1962.

Whitney, Janet. *Abigail Adams.* Boston: Little, Brown and Co., 1947.

MARGARET SHIPPEN ARNOLD

Bradford, Gamaliel. *Wives.* New York: Harper Brothers, 1925.

Ellet, Elizabeth F. *The Queens of American Society.* Philadelphia: Porter and Coates, 1867.

Flexner, James Thomas. *The Traitor and the Spy: Benedict Arnold and John André.* New York: Harcourt Brace and Co., 1953.

Ryerson, A. Egerton. *The Loyalists of America and Their Times, 1620-1816.* 2 vols. New York: Haskell House Pubs., Ltd., 1969.

Van Doren, Carl. *Secret History of the American Revolution.* New York: The Viking Press, Inc., 1941.

Walker, Lewis Burd. "The Wife of Benedict Arnold." *Pennsylvania Magazine of History and Biography* 24 (1900): 257–266, 401–429; 25 (1901): 20–46, 145–190, 289–302, 452–497; 26 (1902): 71–80, 224–244, 322–334, 464–468.

SARAH FRANKLIN BACHE

Gillespie, Mrs. E.D. *A Book of Remembrance.* Philadelphia: J.B. Lippincott Co., 1901.

Labaree, Leonard W., ed. *The Papers of Benjamin Franklin.* New Haven: Yale University Press, 1963.

Van Doren, Carl. *Benjamin Franklin.* New York: The Viking Press, Inc., 1938.

MARGARET CORBIN

Hall, Edward H. *Margaret Corbin.* New York: The American Scenic and Historic Preservation Society, 1932.

Keim, Randolph. "Heroines of the Revolution." *Journal of American History* 22 (1922): 31–35.

LYDIA DARRAGH

Darragh, Henry. "Lydia Darragh of the Revolution." *The Pennsylvania Magazine of History and Biography* 23 (1899): 86–91.

Dexter, Elizabeth A. *Colonial Women of Affairs.* Boston: Houghton Mifflin Co., 1924.

Singer, Kurt D., ed. *Three Thousand Years of Espionage.* Englewood Cliffs, N.J.: Prentice-Hall, Inc. 1948.

Watson, John F. *Annals of Philadelphia and Pennsylvania.* Vol. 2. Philadelphia: Elijah Thomas, 1860.

REBECCA FRANKS

Birmingham, Stephen. *The Grandees.* New York: Harper & Row, Pubs., 1971.

Griswold, Rufus Wilmot. *The Republican Court.* New York: D. Appleton and Co., 1854.

Learsi, Rufus. *The Jew in America: A History.* New York: World Publishing Co., 1954.

"Letter of Miss Rebecca Franks, A." *Pennsylvania Magazine of History and Biography* 16 (1892): 216–218; 23 (1899): 303–309.

Littell, John Stockton, ed. *Graydon's Memoirs of His Own Time.* Philadelphia: Lindsay and Blakiston, 1846.

Memoirs of Lieutenant General Scott, The. Vol. 1. New York: Sheldon and Co., 1864.

Scharf, Thomas, and Westcott, Thompson. *History of Philadelphia.* Vol. 2. Philadelphia: L.H. Everts and Co., 1884.

Simonhoff, Harry. *Jewish Notables in America.* New York: Greenburg, 1956.

Wharton, Anne Hollingsworth. *Through Colonial Doorways.* Philadelphia: J.B. Lippincott Co., 1893.

Wolf, Edward II, and Whiteman, Maxwell. *The History of the Jews in Philadelphia*. Philadelphia: The Jewish Publication Society of America, 1956.

MARY KATHERINE GODDARD

Brigham, Clarence S. *History and Bibliography of American Newspapers, 1690-1820*. Vol. 1. Worcester, Mass.: American Antiquarian Society, 1947.

———. *Journals and Journeymen: A Contribution to the History of Early American Newspapers*. Philadelphia: University of Pennsylvania Press, 1950.

Miner, Ward L. *William Goddard, Newspaperman*. Durham, N.C.: Duke University Press, 1962.

Thomas, Isaiah. *The History of Printing in America, with a Biography of Printers, and an Account of Newspapers*. Vols. I and II. Albany: Joel Munsell, Printer (published under supervision of the American Antiquarian Society), 1874.

Wheeler, Joseph Towne. *The Maryland Press, 1777-1790*. Introduction by Lawrence C.Wroth. Baltimore: The Maryland Historical Society, 1938.

Wroth, Lawrence C. *A History of Printing in Colonial Maryland, 1686-1776*. Baltimore: The Typothetae, 1922.

CATHERINE LITTLEFIELD GREENE

Roelker, William Greene, ed. *Benjamin Franklin and Catherine Ray Greene: Their Correspondence, 1755-1790*. Philadelphia: American Philosophical Society, 1949.

DICEY LANGSTON

Hanaford, Phebe A. *Women of the Century*. Boston: B.B. Russell, 1877.

ANN LEE

Andrews, Edward Deming. *The People Called Shakers: A Search for the Perfect Society.* New York: Oxford University Press, Inc., 1953.

Blinn, Elder Henry C. *The Life and Gospel Experience of Mother Ann Lee.* East Canterbury, N.H.: The Shakers, 1901.

Desroche, Henri. *The American Shakers: From Neo-Christianity to Pre-socialism.* Amherst: The University of Massachusetts Press, 1971.

Evans, Frederick W. *Autobiography of a Shaker and Revelation of the Apocalypse.* Mt. Lebanon, N.Y.: F.W. Evans, 1869.

———. *Shakers.* New York: D. Appleton and Co., 1859.

Joy, Arthur F. *The Queen of the Shakers.* Minneapolis: T.S. Denison, 1960.

Melcher, Marguerite F. *The Shaker Adventure.* Princeton: The Princeton University Press, 1941.

Nordhoff, Charles. *The Communistic Societies of the United States.* New York: Hillary House Publishers, Ltd., 1960.

Noyes, John Humphrey. *History of American Socialisms.* New York: Hillary House Publishers, Ltd., 1961.

Sears, Clara E., ed. *Gleanings from Old Shaker Journals.* Boston: Houghton Mifflin Co., 1916.

Shakers. *A Summary View of the Millennial Church.* 2d ed. Albany. C. Van Benthuysen, 1848.

Shakers. *Testimonies of the Life, Character, Revelations, and Doctrines of Mother Ann Lee.* 2d ed. Albany: Week, Parsons and Co., 1888.

Webber, Everett. *Escape to Utopia.* New York: Hastings House Pubs., Inc., 1959.

Youngs, Benjamin S. *Testimony of Christ's Second Appearing.* Albany: C. Van Benthuysen, 1856.

JANE MECOM

Van Doren, Carl. *Jane Mecom*. New York: The Viking Press, Inc., 1950.

————, ed. *The Letters of Benjamin Franklin and Jane Mecom*. Princeton: Princeton University Press, 1950.

ESTHER DE BERDT REED

Reed, William Bradford. *The Life of Esther De Berdt*. Philadelphia: C. Sherman, 1853.

MARY SLOCUMB

Ellet, Elizabeth F. *The Women of the American Revolution*. 3 vols. Philadelphia: George W. Jacobs and Co., 1900.

Fowler, William W. *Women on the American Frontier*. Hartford: S.S. Scranton and Co., 1878.

Greene, Harry Clinton, and Greene, Mary Wolcott. *Pioneer Mothers of America*. 3 vols. New York: G.P. Putnam's Sons, 1912.

Lefler, Hugh T., and Powell, William S. *Colonial North Carolina: A History*. New York: Charles Scribner's Sons, 1973.

Logan, Mary S. *The Part Taken by Women in American History*. Wilmington, Del.: The Perry-Nalle Publishing Co., 1912.

BARONESS VON RIEDESEL

Blumenthal, Walther Hart. *Women Camp Followers of the American Revolution*. Philadelphia: McManus, 1952.

Pearson, Michael. *The Revolutionary War: An Unbiased Account*. New York: Capricorn, 1973.

Riedesel, Fredericke. *Letters and Journal Relating to the War of the American Revolution and the Capture of the German Troops at Saratoga*. Translated by William L. Stone. Albany: Joel Munsell, 1867.

Tharpe, Louise Hall. *The Baroness and the General*. Boston: Little, Brown and Co., 1962.

Von Eelking, Max, ed. *Memoirs and Letters and Journals of Major-General Riedesel during His Residence in America*. Translated by William L. Stone. Albany: Joel Munsell, 1868.

MERCY OTIS WARREN

Anthony, Katharine. *First Lady of the Revolution: The Life of Mercy Otis Warren*. New York: Doubleday and Co., 1958.

Brown, Alice. *Mercy Warren*. New York: Charles Scribner's Sons, 1903.

Fritz, Jean. *Cast for a Revolution*. Boston: Houghton Mifflin Co., 1972.

Smith, William Raymond. *History as Argument*. The Hague: Mouton and Co., 1966.

Warren, Mercy Otis. *History of the Rise, Progress and Termination of the American Revolution*. Boston: Manning and Loring for E. Larkin, 1805.

Warren-Adams Letters. 2 vols. Boston: Massachusetts Historical Society (Collections), 1917.

MARTHA WASHINGTON

Corbin, John. *The Unknown Washington*. New York: Charles Scribner's Sons, 1930.

Decatur, Stephen, Jr., ed. *The Private Affairs of George Washington, from the Records and Accounts of Tobias Lear, Esquire, His Secretary*. New York: Da Capo Press, 1933.

Donovan, Frank. *The Women in Their Lives*. New York: Dodd, Mead & Co., 1966.

Lossing, Benson J. *Martha Washington*. New York: J.C. Buttre, 1861.

Lowther, Minnie Kendall. *Mount Vernon*. Chicago: John C.Winston, 1930.

Thane, Elswyth. *Washington's Lady.* New York: Dodd, Mead & Co., 1954.

Wecter, Dixon. *The Saga of American Society.* New York: Charles Scribner's Sons, 1937.

Wharton, Anne Hollingsworth. *Colonial Days and Dames.* Philadelphia: J.B. Lippincott, 1895.

———. *Martha Washington.* New York: Charles Scribner's Sons, 1897.

Whitton, Mary Ormsbee. *First First Ladies.* New York: Hastings House Pubs., Ltd., 1948.

PHILLIS WHEATLEY

Brawley, Benjamin. *Early Negro American Writers.* Plainview, N.Y.: Books for Libraries Press, 1935.

Heartman, Charles Frederick, ed. *Phillis Wheatley: Poems and Letters.* Plainview, N.Y.: Books for Libraries Press, 1915.

Katz, William Loren. *Eyewitness: The Negro in American History.* New York: Pitman Publishing Corp., 1967.

Mason, Julian D., Jr., ed. *The Poems of Phillis Wheatley.* Chapel Hill: University of North Carolina Press, 1966.

Renfro, G. Herbert. *Life and Works of Phillis Wheatley.* Plainview, N.Y.: Books for Libraries Press, 1970.

Richmond, M.A. *Bid the Vassal Soar: Interpretive Essays on the Life and Poetry of Phillis Wheatley and George Moses Horton.* Washington, D.C.: Howard University Press, 1974.

Thatcher, B.B. *Memoir of Phillis Wheatley, A Native African and a Slave.* Boston: George W. Light, 1838.

PATIENCE WRIGHT

Einstein, Lewis D. *Divided Loyalties.* London: Cobden-Sanderson, 1933.

Gottesman, Rita S. *The Arts and Crafts in New York, 1726-1776.* New York: The New York Historical Society, 1954.

Hart, C. H. "Patience Wright, Modeller in Wax." *The Connoisseur* 19 (1907): 18–22.

Long, J.C. *Mr. Pitt and America's Birthright.* New York: Frederick A. Stokes Co., 1940.

Schmidt, Minna. *400 Outstanding Women of the World.* Chicago: Minna Schmidt, 1933.

Sellers, Charles C. *Benjamin Franklin in Portraiture.* New Haven: Yale University Press, 1962.

Toynbee, Mrs. Paget, ed. *The Letters of Horace Walpole.* Vol. 8. Oxford: The Clarendon Press, 1904.

Wall, Alexander J. "Wax Portraiture." *The New York Historical Society Quarterly Bulletin.* (April 1925): 3–26.

Watson, Elkanah. *Men and Times of the Revolution.* New York: Dana and Co., 1856.

Whitley, William T. *Artists and Their Friends in England, 1700-1799.* Boston: The Medici Society, 1928.

ADDITIONAL REFERENCES

Adams, Hannah. *A Memoir of Miss Hannah Adams Written by Herself with Additional Notices by a Friend.* Boston: Gray and Bowen, 1832.

Adams, James Truslow, ed. *Album of American History, Colonial Period.* New York: Charles Scribner's Sons, 1944.

Andrist, Ralph K., ed. *The Founding Fathers: George Washington, A Biography in His Own Words.* New York: Newsweek, Inc., 1972.

Barck, Oscar Theodore, and Lefler, Hugh Talmage. *Colonial America.* New York: The Macmillan Co., 1958.

Beard, Mary R. *America through Women's Eyes.* New York: The MacMillan Co., 1934.

Bell, Margaret. *Women of the Wilderness.* New York: E.P. Dutton and Co., 1938.

Bliven, Bruce, Jr. *Under the Guns; New York, 1775-1776.* New York: Harper and Row, Pubs., 1972.

Brodie, Fawn M. *Thomas Jefferson: An Intimate History.* New York: W.W. Norton and Co., 1974.

Carman, Harry J., and Syrett, Harold C. *A History of the American People,* Vol. 1. New York: Alfred A. Knopf, 1952.

Carrington, Henry B. *Battle Maps and Charts of the American Revolution.* New York: Arno Press, 1974.

Cremin, Lawrence A. *American Education: The Colonial Experience, 1607-1786.* New York: Harper & Row, Pubs., 1970.

De Chastellux, Marquis. *Travels in North America.* Chapel Hill: University of North Carolina Press, 1963.

Dorson, Richard M., ed. *American Rebels.* New York: Pantheon, 1953.

Drake, Samuel Adams. *Book of New England Legends and Folk Lore.* Boston: Little, Brown and Co., 1901.

Earle, Alice Morse. *Child Life in Colonial Days.* New York: The MacMillan Co., 1899.

————. *Colonial Dames and Good Wives.* New York: Houghton Mifflin Co., 1901.

————. *Home and Child Life in Colonial Days.* New York: The MacMillan Co., 1908.

Fleming, Thomas J. *The Man from Monticello: An Intimate Life of Thomas Jefferson.* New York: William Morrow & Co., Inc., 1969.

Gerlach, Don R. *Philip Schuyler and the American Revolution in New York, 1733-1777.* Lincoln, Nebraska: University of Nebraska Press, 1964.

Gould, Elizabeth Porter. "Hannah Adams: The Pioneer Woman in American Literature." *The New England Magazine* 10 (1894): 363-369.

Greene, Evarts Boutell. *The Revolutionary Generation .* New York: The Macmillan Co., 1943.

Hall, Gordon Langley. *Mr. Jefferson's Ladies.* Boston: Beacon Press, 1966.

Holliday, Carl. *Woman's Life in Colonial Days.* Boston: The Cornhill Publishing Co., 1922.

Humphrey, Grace. *Women in American History.* Indianapolis: The Bobbs-Merrill Co., Inc., 1919.

Humphreys, Mary Gay. *Catherine Schuyler.* New York: Charles Scribner's Sons, 1897.

————. *Women of Colonial and Revolutionary Times.* New York: Charles Scribner's Sons, 1910.

James, Edward T. and James, Janet W., eds. *Notable American Women, 1607-1950.* 3 vols. Cambridge: The Belknap Press of the Harvard University Press, 1971.

Jameson, John Franklin. *The American Revolution Considered as a Social Movement.* New York: P. Smith, 1950.

Kelly, Joseph J. *Life and Times in Colonial Philadelphia.* Harrisburg, Pa.: Stackpole Books, 1973.

Ketchum, Richard M., ed. *The American Heritage Book of the Revolution.* New York: American Heritage Publishing Co., 1971.

Landis, John B. "Investigation into the American Tradition of a Woman Known as 'Molly Pitcher.'" *The Journal of American History* 5 (1911): 82–96.

Leish, Kenneth W. *The American Heritage Pictorial History of the Presidents of the United States,* Vol. 1. New York: American Heritage Publishing Co., 1968.

Leonard, Eugenie Andruss. *The AmericanWoman in Colonial and Revolutionary Times, 1665-1800.* Philadelphia: The University of Pennsylvania Press, 1962.

Lossing, Benson J. *The Life and Times of Philip Schuyler.* New York: Sheldon and Co., 1860.

Morison, Samuel Eliot. *The Oxford History of the American People.* New York: Oxford University Press, 1965.

"Notes and Queries." *The Pennsylvania Magazine of History and Biography* 3 (1879): 109–110. Pennsylvania Historical Society.

Quincy, Josiah. *Figures of the Past.* Boston: Little, Brown and Co., 1926.

Randolph, Sarah Nicholas. *The Domestic Life of Thomas Jefferson.* New York: Harper Brothers, 1871.

Royall, Anne Newport. *Sketches of History, Life, and Manners in the United States by a Traveller.* New York: Johnson Reprint Corp., 1970.

Spruill, Julia Cherry. *Women's Life and Work in the Southern Colonies.* Chapel Hill: The University of North Carolina Press, 1938.

Sweetser, Kate Dickenson. *Ten American Girls from History.* New York: Harper Brothers, 1917.

Tuckerman, Bayard. *Life of General Philip Schuyler.* New York: Dodd, Mead & Co., 1903.

Vance, Marguerite. *Patsy Jefferson of Monticello.* New York: E. P. Dutton & Co., Inc., 1948.

Walett, Francis G. Introduction to *The Boston Gazette, 1774.* Barre, Mass.: The Imprint Society, 1972.

Warwick, Edward et al. *Early American Dress.* New York: Benjamin Blom, Inc., 1965.

Whitton, Mary Ormsbee. *These Were the Women.* New York: Hastings House Pubs., Inc., 1954.

Winsor, Justin, ed. *The American Revolution.* New York: Sons of Liberty Publications by Land's End Press, 1972.

Woody, Thomas. *History of Women's Education in the United States.* New York: Science Press, 1929.

Index

D

E

F

H

I

J